Release the Seductress Within

✳ ✳ ✳

How to Seduce a Man...and Thrill You Both

Release the Seductress Within

How to Seduce a Man...and Thrill You Both

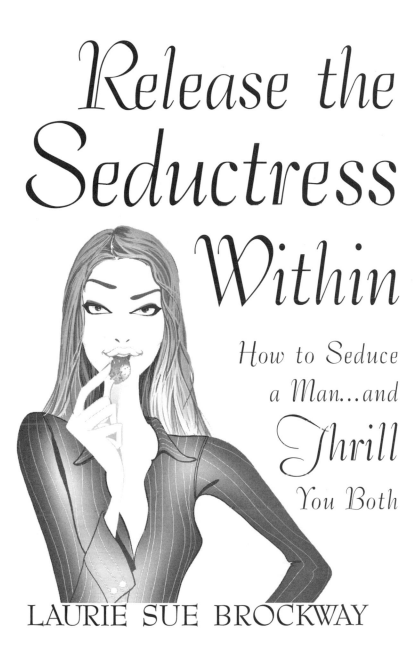

LAURIE SUE BROCKWAY

GRAMERCY BOOKS • NEW YORK

This 2003 edition is published by Gramercy Books, an imprint of Random House
Value Publishing, a division of Random House, Inc., New York, by arrangement with
Kensington Publishing Corp.

Gramercy is a registered trademark and the colophon is a trademark
of Random House, Inc.

Random House
New York • Toronto • London • Sydney • Auckland
www.randomhouse.com

Printed and bound in the United States

Library of Congress Cataloging-in-Publication Data

Brockway, Laurie Sue.
   [How to seduce a man and keep him seduced]
   Release the seductress within : how to seduce a man— and thrill you both /
Laurie Sue Brockway.
      p. cm.
   Originally published: How to seduce a man and keep him seduced / Laurie Sue
Brockway. Secaucus, N.J. : Carol Publishing Group, c1998.
   Includes bibliographical references and index.
   ISBN 0-517-22199-3
      1. Sex instruction for Women. 2. Sexual excitement. 3. Seduction. I. Title.

HQ46.B76 2004
613.9'6'082—dc21

                                                                   2003057280

10 9 8 7 6 5 4 3 2 1

To the goddess in us all

Contents

Preface   ix

Acknowledgments   xv

Test Your Seductress I.Q.   xvii

Introduction   xxiii

Part I   Finding Your Inner Seductress

1   The History and Herstory of Seduction   3

2   Getting to Know Your Inner Seductress   19

3   Unleashing the Sex Goddess   38

4   The Modern Seductress and Her Men   51

Part II   Learning From the Titans of Temptation

5   You've Got to Have Attitude!   63

6   Lessons From the Femme Fatale   69

7   Lessons From the Stripper   76

8   Lessons From the Dominatrix   85

9   Lessons From the Sexpot   97

Part III   *Making It Real*

10 Overcoming Seduction Shyness   107

11 How to Be a Private Dancer   115

12 Hot Talk and Whispers   123

13 Creating the Environment   132

14 Toys "R" Us   143

15 Your Body's Secret Weapon   157

16 Aphrodisiacs, Love Elixirs, and Pleasure Enhancers   162

17 Becoming the Sacred Seductress   172

    In Closing   185

    Appendix: Safe, Responsible Seduction and Sex   188

    Resource Guide   191

    Index   199

Preface

When it comes to seduction, I've been around the block a few times.

My natural curiosity has always drawn me to matters sexual, and my desire to gain wisdom through experience has led me to try many things. I can honestly say that from stripping for an audience of one to becoming a sacred seductress, I have personally tried almost everything I recommend to you in this book.

My deep interest in sexual self-esteem and my desire to free my own erotic expression has taken me down many paths. As a single woman, I lived much of my adult life in a way that this culture often associates with a certain kind of bachelor—I went after the men and the experiences I wanted, and I was not shy about pursuing sex. That is how I honed my skills as a seductress: I saw something I wanted and figured out how to get it. Seduction was a way of attracting men and communicating.

My approach didn't always work. I was rejected and ignored. I was passed over for prettier women many times. But I never stopped trying—I kept taking risks. To me, every step of the journey was a lesson. When I resisted what life was trying to teach me, I felt pain; when I paid attention to and learned from the secret messages embedded in every experience, life flowed and I grew.

Finally, I came to a point in my own evolution where I wanted more than just the sexual challenge. I longed to learn about the sacred secrets of sexuality and to connect with a man in a way that transcended the boudoir. That is where my path led me...and I had fun every step of the way.

How It Began

I was never "traditionally" beautiful. I always carried extra weight, so I had to find a way to get male attention in a culture that preferred slim, beautiful women with perfect, pert breasts as opposed to a woman formed more like the great earth goddess Gaia, with a round belly and pendulous breasts—like me.

I had a few strikes against me from the start. My mother had a weight problem all her life, and my tendency toward chubbiness was a big issue in my family. My mom, my grandmother, and Lord knows how many people who said, "You have such a pretty face, but..." drove home the point at a young age: *I wasn't thin enough.* That translated to *I wasn't good enough.* I am not exaggerating when I say it scarred my self-esteem, and I still haven't completely healed from the pain of feeling so unattractive and unworthy because my body is not ideal.

My father began drinking when I was eight and separated from my mother when I was eighteen. The disease of alcoholism made him a bad model of male behavior during my formative years, and his leaving home was a major abandonment in my life. Those two aspects of my childhood were the source of the problems I was to face with men, the saddest being the belief that I carried for so long: *My father left me and this must mean I am unlovable.*

I've had enough therapy and have done enough inner work to

have learned that it was my inner child who believed I was unworthy. But before I learned to pay more attention to my inner goddess, I reacted to the belief that I was unworthy and unlovable. I had to think of a way to become worthier and to get attention from men, so I became sexy, seductive, and smart.

I figured if I couldn't catch a guy's attention with my looks, I'd either grab him with my sexually open attitude or I'd blow him away in the bedroom. The good part was that I spent a lot of time developing an interesting life so that I'd have some fun stories to fall back on. In the process, I became a woman of substance.

The not-so-great part was that in my early years as an evolving seductress, I was coming from a place of need for love (*my father left me and therefore I must not be lovable*) and fear of not being accepted (*I am not thin enough, therefore I am not worthy enough*), so I sold myself short with guys a number of times before I realized my true power as a seductress. I think we all grow by giving away our power and trying to reclaim it. When I finally found the goddess who dwelled within me, I did everything I could think of to bring her out to play. I must have been on the right track because, no matter what my weight was, I have had men around me throughout my adult life. Beyond the male attention and the sensual exchange, I literally built the latter part of my career on seduction and understanding the components of male-female dynamics.

From being a teenage chubbette who sat back and watched in painful silence as all the cute guys chose my prettier, thinner girlfriends (although they always liked me as a "buddy"), I have gone on to become someone who is sexually confident and professionally experienced enough to write a book on the topic! I'd say I have turned myself into a seductress success story. And that's why I know *you* can be a seductress success story too.

You can start out shy and demure, fat or skinny, too tall or too flat, with features that aren't quite right or body parts that you'd like to hide, and yet, with determination and spirit, you can find the seductress who lives within you. The sex goddess in all of us is beautiful and bold. I still have to remind myself not to listen to anyone who tells me anything different!

Working Seduction

I had so much fun with seduction that I turned it into a job! In 1990, after twelve years as a general assignment reporter who specialized in sexuality whenever possible, I began editing sex books. I would insert steamy scenes to make existing manuscripts even hotter. Next, I began penning erotica from the female perspective that featured savvy, sexy career women who utilized their powers of seduction to have wonderful, sensual relations with men. I wrote five books that led me on one adventure after another. All of life felt like a big, ongoing date in which I was the queen of seduction.

In the early 1990s, I publicly took a stand for empowering women to express their seductive natures and own their sensuality, and my work caught the eye of the folks at *Playgirl*. They asked me to come on as editor-in-chief. When I was in college, I used to ask men to pose for me for a study of male nudes that I was doing for a photography class (yeah, right!)—and now here I was, editor of the nation's only sex magazine for women! The job was an erotic picnic. I had permission to be seductive and to express my sensual nature, and that license helped me develop the confidence to communicate with total openness about sexuality. As for all those gorgeous, hot-bodied men who would line up to get to know me...that was not a bad perk either. Having access to men of such physical beauty cured me of being intimidated by hunks.

During my reign at *Playgirl*, I had the opportunity to experience myriad assignments that brought out my inner seductress. I took dominatrix lessons. I hired a nude handyman to put up shelves as I watched. I spent a night with a hired gigolo who attended to my pleasure for almost twenty-four hours. I dated a highly sexed gynecologist who helped me discover my G spot. I had a lot of fun, and I incorporated every experience into my seductress repertoire. My work gave me the best seduction lines on the planet:

"Hi. I'm the editor in chief of *Playgirl* magazine."

"Hi. I write erotic books."

"Hi. I've taken dominatrix lessons and know how to use a whip."

I began to get a real kick out of my own power as a seductress, for any of these introuctions had the same effect as putting my hands down a guy's pants. It made men hot and it got me excited to see that simply by exploring my own passions, I was a turn-on to men.

Although most women will not use the same lines that I have (but hey, go ahead and make up some new ones for yourself), any woman can learn to communicate in a way that arouses a man's interest and entices him. I believe the things that turn us on most are the things that make us most attractive to others. That is why seduction is an inside job; being a seductress means drawing on the passion and desire within you.

Women who know how to bring pleasure to themselves are often the best seducers. Seduction used to mean "man-pleasing"—luring a guy in and trying to get him to stay. I think modern sex goddesses now understand that the spirit of seduction is being true to yourself—pleasing yourself first and then sharing it with the right person.

When I learned that lesson, my career shifted gears. I was done with solo explorations in sex. My inner sex goddess gently steered me along another path. I became more interested in reporting on and experiencing spiritual aspects of sexuality and relationships. I wanted to take seduction to a higher level. Soon enough, the right person came along and the tone of my exploration changed. I had a playmate! I thought having a partner would be limiting, but now I know that when you seduce the right man, life becomes more expansive and expressive.

When you are with a man you want to keep under your spell, you set your inner seductress free in a relationship in which she is honored and respected. Some people call this love!

Acknowledgments

The writing of this book coincided with a time of total transformation in my life. My father became very ill in January 1997 and died that April. It was a devastating loss. My health—emotional and physical—took the hit.

Because of my father's death this is a very different book than the one I intended to write. While writing it, my life experience was so far out of the realm of "seduction" that I had to reach deep into my heart for the story I wanted to tell. My inner seductress rose through the pain to help me write this book.

I have to thank my dad for putting me on a path that led me beyond the *surface* of seduction, to the *spirit* of seduction.

I also have to thank my editor, Carrie Nichols Cantor, of Carol Publishing Group, for demonstrating patience and understanding beyond reason, and for helping me take this book in a direction that is far more meaningful than, as they say in *Damn Yankees,* "a standard seduction."

I thank my agent, Laura Tucker, for asking me to write this book and my friend Susan Crain Bakos for networking me to her. Thanks also to my sister, Nikki Lynne Fiske, the elementary school teacher, and my mom, Shirley Brockway, the grammar whiz, who helped with some last-minute copyediting as my sister Rikki Rosenberg assured me that "everything will work out."

My most understanding family member was my six-year-old

son, Alexander Kent Garrett, who for many months saw his mom in one of two positions: crying about Grandpa or huddled over the computer working. I hope I can make it up to him.

I thank all my goddess friends who so generously contributed to me and the book with information, insights, and prayers. And I thank the many experts and sources whom I interviewed for *Playgirl* and *Single Living* who provided insight for this book.

Last but not least, a thank-you to Dr. Richard A. Cohn, who through his love, wisdom, and expertise contributed to this project in many ways.

Test Your Seductress I.Q.

It takes one to know one. How much do you know about seductresses and seduction through the ages?

1. Cleopatra is famous for seducing men with her:
   a. Hairstyle
   b. Dancing girls
   c. Scents and passion potions
   d. Eyes

2. A dominatrix is a:
   a. Woman who assists with childbirth
   b. Mistress
   c. Dominican nun
   d. A dominoes player

3. Lolita, the literary character, is:
   a. An exotic dancer from Long Island
   b. Young and irresistible to an older man
   c. A baby-sitter
   d. The spinster sister of the author Vladimir Nabokov

4. A female who enjoys chasing men for sport, pleasure, and sexual satisfaction is a:
   a. Black widow spider

    b. Tomboy
    c. Athlete
    d. Huntress

5. Mercilessly seducing and using men is the sport of:
    a. The preying mantis
    b. Mae West
    c. The femme fatale
    d. Gidget

6. The Sacred Prostitute is:
    a. A friend of Eddie Murphy's
    b. An older hooker
    c. A brothel in Nevada
    d. A revered woman who initiates and heals men through sex

7. Mae West was most likely considered a sexpot because she:
    a. Had blond hair and a round butt
    b. Did a movie with W. C. Fields
    c. Had attitude!
    d. Wore a lot of robes in movies

8. Which movie title best relays Ann-Margret's sultry girl-next-door/-vixen image:
    a. *Kitten With a Whip*
    b. *Bye-Bye Birdie*
    c. *Viva, Las Vegas*
    d. *Grumpy Old Men*

9. The best place to go to watch an exotic dancer in action is:
    a. The Caribbean
    b. A strip club
    c. Milan
    d. The Big Island of Hawaii

10. To the seductress, role playing and acting out means:

    a. Working through issues in therapy
    b. Performing on stage
    c. Safely living out a few favorite fantasies/creating sexual theater
    b. Talking to pillows and pretending they're your parents

11. What is the ancient, women-centered sexual practice that focuses on the female's "sacred spot"?
    a. Tantra
    b. Kama Sutra
    c. Buddhist Romance
    d. Wild love

12. An herbal aphrodisiac is a:
    a. Shampoo
    b. Laxative
    c. Love stimulant
    d. New restaurant

13. In Greek mythology, the goddess of sex and love is:
    a. Vampira
    b. Eros
    c. Aphrodite
    d. Hera

14. Throughout history, women have utilized their sexual charm and know-how to seduce men. One of the most effective methods is:
    a. Greeting him naked at the door
    b. Cooking for him
    c. Working for the same company
    d. Letting him chase, get a taste, and come back for more

15. The *last* thing a man wants to hear as you seduce him is:
    a. You're pregnant with his child
    b. Sports scores

c. His mother's voice

d. Complaints of any kind, especially about his sexual skill

Answers

1. c. In addition to her guts and guile, Cleopatra is famous for her use of scents and love elixirs to seal her seductions.

2. b. A dominatrix is a sexually dominant female who is respectfully addressed as "Mistress."

3. b. Lolita is the name of the famous young female whom Humbert Humbert found irresistible in the Vladimir Nabokov novel by the same name. She is the prototype of the nubile, young thing.

4. d. Sexually open women who pursue sex in a manner usually equated with single men seem to relish being thought of as a "Huntress."

5. c. Femme fatales are most famous for hooking men in for the sole purpose of using them to accomplish an awful, evil deed. In Hollywood movies they are portrayed as beautiful but heartless, cold-blooded killers; in history, some femme fatales, such as Mata Hari, at least had a cause.

6. d. The sacred prostitutes of ancient times served to heal and initiate men to the way of the goddess. Today, they have lots of fun doing it!

7. c. While Mae West had the kind of bust and butt that drove vaudevillians wild, it was her sassy, sexually playful attitude that made her a sexpot!

8. a. Ann-Margret starred in all those films, but *Kitten With A Whip* best describes her image: a sweet, purring, good girl (kitten) whose molten sensuality smolders beneath (whip).

9. b. Exotic dancer is the politically correct term for a stripper.

10. c. One of the great joys of a budding seductress is the opportunity to live out some fantasies in the privacy of her own, self-created "sexual theater"!
11. a. The primary focus of Tantric sex, which is a form of what is known as "esoteric" or "sacred" sexual practice, is a spiritual connection; however, one of the ways to access it is through tender loving tribute paid to the female's "sacred spot," also known as the G spot.
12. c. There is an array of herbal aphrodisiacs which help to create erotic stimulation, sensual excitement, and blood flow to all the right places.
13. c. Aphrodite is the Greek goddess of love and sex. The Romans called her Venus.
14. d. Throughout the ages, letting the man chase you, or at least letting him think he is, still seems to be one of the most seductive activities known to men.
15. d. The most certain sabotage of a seduction in progress is complaining. Save it. There's a time and a place.

Tally Your Score

Study, girlfriend: If you got five or less answers right, you need this book…bad!

Work it: If you got between six and ten answers right, you are on track and would benefit from learning a few more tricks and trying them out.

You go, girl: If you were correct on between eleven and fifteen answers, you come to this book with a high Seductress I.Q. With commitment, enhanced knowledge and practice, you too can *seduce your man and keep him under your spell.*

Note: Don't worry about your score. Everyone has to start somewhere!

Introduction

The average man is more interested in a woman who
is interested in him than he is in a woman—any
woman—with beautiful legs.

—Marlene Dietrich

There are many directions a woman can take when it comes to
seducing a man and keeping him seduced. The range is as huge as
life itself. You can demurely invite and suggest, manipulate and
cajole, aggressively chase and overwhelm a man. You can knock a
guy's socks off by showing your wild-woman self. You can cook,
bake, and win him over with aphrodisiacal dinners. You can smile,
bat your eyelashes, and drop hankies. The right strategy might
even depend on your mood and his. There simply is no "right"
way to seduce a guy.

But I truly believe there is only one way a woman can set out to
accomplish her seduction goals *and* be true to herself. That is to
discover her inner seductress, to get to know the sex goddess
within, and from that vantage point decide which approach
(including props and accessories) is most appropriate and
meaningful to her.

Once you discover the seductress who dwells within, you can
seduce anyone. You are likely to find that once a woman has

tapped into her inner sex goddess, all she has to do is show interest in a man to attract his attention.

The aim of this book is to give any woman the key to becoming a successful seductress by introducing her to the beautiful female spirit within her. A woman at any starting point, of any age, shape, or size, can access the tools necessary to seduce a man and keep him under her spell. Don't be surprised to find that the most important tool is your attitude and the willingness to launch seduction from within your own heart and soul!

The Sex Goddess in You

Being seductive isn't about the *way* you look, it's about the way you think or feel you look. Poor self-esteem is an epidemic in this country, and women often grow up feeling inferior because they do not look like the models and actresses who dominate the pages of magazines. Some women develop a distorted self-image. You would be amazed at how your feelings are mirrored by your look and demeanor. That is why the first part of this book is devoted to helping you meet your inner seductress. As you go beyond the surface of your ideas, beliefs, and fears about your sexuality and ability to seduce, you'll begin to identify your self-image challenges and rise above any negative feelings you might have about your own flesh.

As you become un-brainwashed about beauty, you will discover the truth about seduction: an effective true seductress expresses and exudes sexuality beyond the skin she is in or the outfit she is wearing. It really doesn't matter whether you are skinny or chunky, short or tall, mousy or pushy, quick to learn or slow to start. What matters is your willingness to go for it, regardless of some of the beliefs you may have about your ability to be seductive. What matters is that you create a vision of who you want to become as a seductress and adhere to it, as if you are living out a fantasy. From that perspective, you will follow a path that feels right to you personally and the right men will be drawn to you like moths to a flame.

Becoming a conscious seductress—one who pays attention to her life, her desires, her vision for the future—will enable you to put your focus in the right place. This book will address letting go of old beliefs—whether they be *I'm not sexy enough* or *I'm too shy*—and focusing on the positive. The best way to start a chain reaction of empowerment in a woman is to get her to stop focusing on the parts of her body or sexuality that she doesn't like.

Yasmine Bleeth, an extraordinary beauty who came to international prominence in *Baywatch,* is a woman you would never expect to have a bad hair day. She told me a key to her good self-esteem was not trying to compare herself to other people! "That's really important...even for me," she said. "You can't go around comparing yourself to someone who's taller, thinner, has bigger boobs or better hips. Your have to just try to feel good about yourself and do whatever it takes to make yourself feel good."

Focusing on aspects of yourself that you already like will help you have better self-appreciation. Perhaps you have gorgeous eyes, a dazzling smile, beautiful breasts, perfect teeth, or sexy toes...use those aspects of yourself to begin to see the beauty that lies beneath the surface. "I think people should show off their best asset, whatever it is," says Bleeth. "Everyone has something that's beautiful. Women worry too much about the way they look. I really believe that beauty comes in all shapes and sizes. It's just that sometimes we see ourselves in a certain way, and imagine that's how others see us."

Dating coach Myreah Moore, author of *My, My, My...Dating in the 1990s,* adds that the most successful seductress is a woman who is "in her glory" as a woman. "It's not in a woman's physical makeup," she says. "It doesn't matter what size or shape you are. What matters is that you love yourself and honor yourself. I think women should focus on the most profound aspects of themselves—from their hearts and minds to their eyes or fingernails—because those are the parts that attract people to them."

Communication Is Key

One of the most important points this book will make about seduction is that it's all about communication—not performance and cute outfits. Communication can include enticing, tantalizing, arousing, and even performing for your man... but it's not about doing something to someone, it's about doing something with someone. If the object of your seduction is not a full participant, attempts to seduce will become manipulation. Seduction is supposed to be fun and exciting—not hard work.

While there are many tips and ideas for being sexy and seductive, the larger focus is on tapping into your feelings and gradually bringing them out. Since seduction is about communication, try to imagine what happens when you expand your ability to consciously communicate with words, actions, and body language. It will be like learning a whole new language. Every time you practice and take a step beyond where you started, you expand your comfort zone, and each time your comfort zone gets bigger, your life gets richer and fuller. You will find that as your talents evolve in the arena of love, sex, and romance, other parts of your life will begin to open up as well.

One of the ways you can begin to expand your comfort level is by finding role models—women who express themselves in ways that you would like to emulate. In the section "Titans of Temptation," there are suggested movies to view and seductress assignments to try out, but you can begin your fact-finding mission immediately by noticing the way women walk, talk, and maintain eye contact.

You don't have to look for movie stars and strippers as role models. Look around at women like you—with similar body types, backgrounds, haircuts, fashion sense—who do the kind of things you would like to do. Just notice how they do it and try it sometime. Perhaps that waitress runs her fingers through her hair a certain way, or a friend at work has a way of smiling that is really attractive. Emulating pleasant traits in others is not about being a copycat; it is about incorporating new modes of self-expression into your life.

Keeping Him Seduced

While women have searched the globe for ways to keep men interested and engaged in a relationship, the truth is that none of us can hold a man who doesn't want to be held. The more you get in touch with your inner goddess, the less need you will have for men who require a lot of work.

Seductresses throughout history, whom you will meet in the coming chapters, have used all sorts of techniques for tempting men. You will probably want to give some of them a try. It is important to maintain a clear vision of the relationship you desire in your future as you envision the seductress you want to become, because you want to make sure you get the right man under your spell.

While the idea of keeping a man under your spell might seem like some kind of magic, I believe you will find it has more to do with freedom and love. The key is in your hands: You become all the woman you can be, and the rest will fall into place.

Remember the film *Field of Dreams,* where Kevin Costner kept hearing "Build it and they will come?" I believe a similar premise is at work here. Build your own life, and your beloved will find you are already a complete woman when he steps in to join you.

PART I ❤

Finding Your Inner Seductress

1

The History and Herstory of Seduction

Since the dawn of time, women have been seducing men. Perhaps the first seduction took place the moment Eve and Adam bit into the apple in the Garden of Eden. From the very start, one gets the sense that a man (even the first man) could not refuse the urging of a naked woman: "Oh, Adam...just one, tiny, teenie-weenie, little bite."

The most prevalent spin on seductresses through history is that they seem to be...bad. Oh, so bad! The seductress is also usually a woman of power—a power that relies heavily on or is intensified by womanly ways and wiles—who knows her own mind and understands the nature of the male. Because of this understanding, she often demonstrates the ability to control men subtly, and not so subtly, through her sexuality.

While the seductress has often been viewed through the ages as a fallen woman, it's time to reframe that view and recognize the naturalness and appropriateness of such a role falling to women.

There are thousands of cases in point—in the Bible, history books, literature, the movies, and real life—that confirm the following: Most men want to be seduced, and women are the best seducers on the planet. (And if you include sci-fi sexpots like Barbarella—portrayed by Jane Fonda—you can make that in the galaxy!)

Throughout history men have been led to temptation, spun into ecstasy by the notion of pleasing a woman and being rewarded with her love and affection. For some men, temptation has led to a gloriously open heart and titillation of the loins, but for others it has led to self-destruction. At the very least, a bold and skillful seductress has more than once been powerful enough to weave some very sticky political webs, initiate a war, or bring down a leader. The parable of Adam and Eve and the concept of original sin are the model. Samson and Delilah, Cleopatra and Caesar, and even Pocahontas and John Smith are love matches that involved a woman who in some way unraveled a man or controlled his destiny through seduction. But seductresses, more often than not, take no prisoners; they merely know how to extend an invitation to a man in such a way that he surrenders to passion.

So who says women are the weaker sex? I think the female's ability to turn a man to putty in her hands has been underutilized, underrated, and misunderstood. It's time we celebrate the true power of the female and recognize the importance of being a seductress. Seductresses have changed the course of history. We may not all have such lofty plans—perhaps a hot Saturday night will do—yet it is useful to take a peek at some of our heroines' time-tested techniques, tools, and tricks of the trade. Many of the seductresses throughout history were quite creative and bold, and many of their ideas have modern applications. For example:

- ♥ Cleopatra, Egyptian Queen of the Nile, used bold theatrics to get Julius Caesar's attention by having herself rolled naked in a rug and delivered to his chamber. To get Mark Antony, she sailed into Rome on a glitzy party ship with sails saturated by the sensual scent of Jasmine. It was so rich and entertaining that he could not resist going after his best friend's former lover. When it came to keeping a man under her spell, she was known for the use of aromatics and potions. Cleopatra's fruity love elixir was said to stir the loins of the lowliest servants, who, after sipping the concoction, would pledge loyalty.

- Josephine kept her beloved conqueror, Napoleon Bonaparte, hooked during the French Empire by giving him something most modern women would fear is socially incorrect, not to mention unhygienic: her unbathed body, with all its natural scents. Legend has it she would not bathe for a week before his return from battle because he adored her natural aromas. She'd anoint herself with violets, mixing that aphrodisiacal scent with her natural pheromones. When sending him off to war again, she'd make sure the scent of violets went with him so that he would go crazy for her while away from home.

- Mata Hari knew in war-torn France what women have known for centuries: dance is a way to express the erotic, and dancers have the ability to titillate the imagination and to tantalize men. She captured the attentions of many, not just with beauty but also with charm and her ability to lure men by using her gift for entertaining them. In her heyday, her stardom was an aphrodisiac few men could ignore. The fact that she could be like an ice queen, removed and distant (just like the actress Greta Garbo, who portrayed her in the classic 1932 film *Mata Hari*) added to her allure. Of course, Mata Hari was alleged to be a spy, and an appearance before a firing squad sealed her fate. Yet she was a seductress extraordinaire who turned espionage into an art form, and knew how to enlist powerful men to help her cause.

- Actress Virginia Hill apparently understood that one way to a man's heart was to be uninterested, unavailable, and involved with someone else! It worked on famed gangster Bugsy Siegel, who pursued the sexy Miss Hill with pitbull tenacity. Once he did win her over, he wooed her with Hollywood contacts and charm; she became a trustworthy companion, seducing him yet again by giving him what most men need from a woman: acknowledgment and validation. She believed in him—particularly his cockamamie plan to build a city in the heart of the desert. They called it Las Vegas! (Perhaps Annette Bening, who portrayed Hill in the movie *Bugsy,* knew a little something about the allure of the hard-to-win woman: she ended up marrying the star, Warren Beatty. She said his legendary liaisons with leading ladies did not faze her, and his looks didn't make her want to jump him.)

💗 And let's not forget about Madonna, the end-of-the-millennium answer to ripping the lid off female inhibition and giving women permission to be boldly erotic, exotic, and their own person. In some ways, she is the ultimate seductress—the one a man can't stop, have, or control—and the ultimate role model for the modern seductress. While you can see the roots of Madonna's sexual aura in blond bombshells such as Marilyn Monroe, Jayne Mansfield, and Mae West, her in-your-face style is her own creation. While not every female aspires to put on such a show of it, Madonna embodies entitlement and exudes confidence—two keys to seductress success. Madonna once said this about being a sex symbol: "I guess I would be perceived as that because I have a typically voluptuous body, because the way I dress accents my femininity, and because a lot of what I am about is just expressing sexual desire and not really caring what people think about it."

Bad Girls or Miss-Understoods?

Seduction has always been something at which females could excel. Historically, men were far more physically, politically, socially, and financially dominant than women, and sex was one of the few domains left for females. Women, for many generations, relied on sexual manipulation as a survival mechanism—simple stuff like "I'll give you sex if you give me a pretty new toga...a shiny chariot...a fur coat...food for my children," and so forth. Sex, for many women, was simply a means to an end.

Then there were the conscious seductresses who understood that sexual savvy, erotic acumen, and an understanding of how to properly please and manage a man are good skills to have. Think back to the fifties: a pretty face, nice boobs in a tight sweater, and the ability to type sixty-five words per minute helped, yet management of the male was the ultimate seductress skill. It was perfectly natural for a woman to lure a man in and then take charge of his life, all the while making him feel as if he were the boss!

In simple terms, managing a man means taking the initiative and making things happen without threatening a man's masculinity. In fact, seductresses of the highest order understand that the key to keeping a man under their spell is to enhance his masculine pride by making him feel he is well worth a woman's time, energy, and creativity!

Cleopatra was a queen, but she wasn't too high and mighty to stroke Caesar's male ego, along with certain body parts (remember their first meeting). She was not, according to historical data and drawings, a great beauty, but she knew how to get into the worlds of great men by seducing their minds and all their senses. Perhaps she was simply the ultimate woman she could be and, in her presence, men felt honored, appreciated, or simply unable to resist!

Topping From Below

Today, in the world of D&S (Dominance and Submission—a term that is often used interchangably with S & M, sadomasochism, and B&D, bondage and discipline), they call a partner who is considered to be submissive a "bottom." The dominant partner is a "top." In many cases, it is actually the submissive partner who controls the relationship. It's called "topping from below."

The traditional male–female dynamics of this culture—i.e., "You Jane, me Tarzan"—have led many women to realize that topping from below is perhaps the most prevalent, time-tested, successful way to seduce. It's likely we've all done it without thinking twice because, in the flow of life. as we know it in this culture, it is often the natural order of things. It means simply that the submissive partner "manages" the relationship in such a way that the dominant partner is always made to feel masterful and yet is strongly influenced by the desires of the submissive partner. Just look at the traditional male-female relationship: He earns the money, she spends it. He is the "hunter" and she is the "gatherer." The truth is, wanting to fulfill the woman's needs gives the man reason to hunt. The woman who lets a man fulfill her needs has a mighty power, for she is in fact allowing a man to do something he very naturally wants to do—make his woman happy.

Sacred Seduction

What many people do not realize is that five thousand years ago, God was viewed as a female, the Divine Mother. Men worshipped Goddess as a deity, and thus in many cultures females were honored and their sexuality was considered sacred.

"Predating Christianity by thousands of years, Goddess worship revered and valued the feminine principle," writes Elisabeth Brooke, in her chapter on "Goddess as Healer" in *Medicine Woman*. "Early culture [was] very much the product of the feminine. Woman was seen as the embodiment of power and was associated with the abundance of the Earth and life itself."

Because of their high standing in some ancient societies,

women not only had permission to seduce and to serve men through their seductive abilities, it was part of their responsibility to initiate men. When a revered woman allowed a man to enter her through intercourse, it was believed she was granting him entrance to the path of enlightenment. It was considered a holy rite of passage. Ancients who sought personal attainment of divinity believed union with the female was the closest a man could get to God.

Many cultures honored the "Sacred Prostitute"—women, often from well-to-do families, who chose independence and self-ownership. They served at the pleasure of the goddess, in the temples, utilizing their prowess to heal men. A holy seductress of that kind was considered a high priestess. "Priestesses took their homes in the temples, devoting their lives and bodies to the Great Goddess," says Diana Rose Heartwoman, who wrote "Musing on the Sacred Whore," for *Ecstasy: The Journal of Divine Eroticism* (vol. 2, no. 3). "Male devotees would give just about anything to be initiated by a Sacred Whore, and in doing so, they attained the power of the Great Goddess, as well as contact with what might be called the higher self or divinity within."

"To have intercourse with a prostitute is a virtue that takes away sin," or so says an ancient Indian temple hymn. The *Encyclopedia of Erotic Wisdom* notes, "It is no exaggeration to say that sacred prostitution—also called religious, ritual, or temple prostitution—was known to cultures on each and every continent."

Back to the Goddess?

It has been about five millennia since the demise of goddess worship. Today, we are witnessing a resurgence of the search for the sacred relationship and the belief that woman initiates man to pleasures that are both healthy and holy. It took a full-scale women's movement and sexual revolution to begin to regenerate the goddess in women, so that they could fully revel in their own sexual-sensual self-expression. Conservative forces of this nation have worked fiercely to shut down that expression because a woman in touch with her inner seductress is a force to be reckoned with and that jeopardizes the status quo. As author Erica Jong told me not long ago, "Being in touch with your own sexuality puts you in touch with your own liberty, your own sense of freedom, power, and self-empowerment." While this is not a state of being that modern culture as a whole has supported a woman in achieving, there are clearly many women who are choosing to tap into their inner prowess and express the holy seductress within.

In Public View

Prior to the women's revolution that liberated women from traditional models, there were seductresses who expressed themselves in a vocal and public way—such as entertainer Josephine Baker, actress Mae West, and author Anaïs Nin—but they were clearly a minority. One of this culture's ultimate icons of seduction was Marilyn Monroe, who stood for female sensual expression and vast seductive power over men. Sadly, she was all sex goddess on the outside, yet too fragile on the inside to own up to her power to express her inner seductress.

Marilyn Monroe was a product of a time in which most female sexuality was based on a woman's ability to attract a man's attention, entice him, tempt him, charm him, and turn him on—which is great stuff—but the spin on women and sex was almost always geared toward man-pleasing. In our time, men still very much appreciate beauty, but they prefer being with a woman who is fully present, enjoying herself, and actively partaking in any sexual exchange. While a man may settle for having it *done to him,* he is more desirous of sharing a moment of sexual possession and power with a female.

What Do You Call a Woman Who...?

Although women today can apply many time-tested seduction secrets in a sex-positive and healthy way, most seductresses throughout history have not had the advantage of being held up as role models. Few people had ever heard of the Sacred Prostitute, and most seductresses were not recognized for the true power of their passion and their willingness to express it.

From the beginning of time, most seductresses were defined as harlots, whores, wenches, witches, bitches, and femmes fatales. Today we have politically correct terms that apply to modern seductresses, such as sex-positive woman, sexual dominant, fantasy engineer, and ladies who love sex; or we call them babes, sirens, sexpots, or enchantresses. And those are compliments indeed, a vast improvement over less honorable terminology.

Thinking of a woman who enjoys sensual self-expression and seduction as a bimbo, nympho, or sex-crazed maneater is an attitude that reflects the old double standard: Casanova has always been considered a great lover, while females with similar appetites and powers of persuasion are looked upon as fallen women. Madonna, the singing siren, summed it up this way: "Sexy boys never get bad press."

Mary Magdalene is a good example. For eons she was remembered as a prostitute, a bad girl transformed only by the love of Christ and only because He forgave her sins. Unanswered questions about her story inspired an investigation that led V.I.E.W. Video in New York to the creation of the documentary *Mary Magdalene: An Intimate Portrait,* in which many modern scholars and religious leaders who were interviewed say that they believe she was actually responsible for keeping Christ's crusade alive. She is cited as a powerful, passionate, historical figure who appears more prominently in the Bible than any other female. In the context of seductress, perhaps Magdalene's ultimate seduction was her belief in Him and all He stood for. Believing in a man and validating his point of view continues to be one of the greatest secrets of seduction.

If You've Got It, Flaunt It

In an episode of the popular situation comedy *Home Improvement,* the character of the wife and mother, portrayed by actress Patricia Richards, once said, "I don't approve of women who flaunt their sexuality to get what they want...I know, because I do that at least three times a day!"

One way to honor the seductress in every woman is to acknowledge that she exists in us all and to reframe our idea of "flaunting what we have." How about characterizing sensual expression as a form of communication that women can be quite good at and men are quite amenable to?

Consider this: Beneath the modern exterior of civilized men and women we are beings ruled by primal urges, the collective unconscious, and the drives of our own subconscious minds. Men are genetically programmed to want to procreate with as many females as humanly possible—hence, the frequency of erections, the inability to stop thinking about sex, and the lifelong yearning for nubile twenty-one-year-olds—and women are genetically engineered to allure the man so that he will bring his seed to her and then stick around to hunt for food, build shelter, and care for her and all their offspring.

In the heyday of feminism, housewifery and motherhood were considered a sublimation of female power; yet many women today understand it is a form of expressing female power—albeit not the only form. Most humans are driven quite naturally by the urge to mate. In nature's dance between the sexes, it is the female who sets the tone and pace and gives permission to continue the dance. Throughout the animal and human kingdoms it is the female who carries the dance card, and it is the male who has to sign on or lose out. In nature's scheme of things, the role of seduction quite naturally falls to the female.

The Ball Is in Your Court

The fact that a woman often longs to be connected to a man through marriage, companionship, or partnership shows that mating is an impulse that cannot be denied. As much as we sometimes don't want to be bothered by men, we are often bothered without them—hot and bothered, that is. Seduction is a way for the female to get her needs met and keep her hormones in balance. As Elizabeth Blackwell, the first woman in the United States to obtain a medical degree, once put it, "The total deprivation of sex produces irritability." The title of director Spike Lee's first feature film sums it up: *She's Gotta Have It!*

It's important to remember that historically, biologically, and psychically, the ball is in the woman's court. Old-fashioned as it may seem, biological reality points again to what history has demonstrated: men court, women seduce. A man can only court a woman who is willing to have him. A woman, however, can seduce whomever she chooses. Thus, tapping into your own inner seductress equals tapping into personal power. And tapping into personal power can equal seducing the man of your choice!

This explains the hold that sexy sirens, strippers, and sex workers have over men. Women who can be paid for sensual arousal are the average man's only hope for domination over women. Paying for service rendered is the only way to guarantee the power to select and the safety to live out the fantasy. Yet our own husbands, boyfriends, brothers, and fathers—and those that came before them—are torn between the need for sexual stimulation and release and the social demand to be upstanding citizens. "There is a glaring contradiction between natural demands and certain social institutions," writes Wilhelm Reich in his classic *The Function of the Orgasm.* "Man is immersed in this contradiction...the human structure is molded in this struggle."

Because men yearn for sexual freedom, choice, and abundance, they have historically set up cultures where they could claim it: sultans and their harems, the Romans and their orgies, the polygamists and their multiple brides. When religious systems touted celibacy and monogamy and the culture at large would not support rampant sexual expression, men set up a structure in which they could get it on the sly—from hookers, lap dancers, strippers, and mistresses.

Today, the United States is home to a multibillion-dollar sex industry. Even though right-wing zealots fight it and deny it, you have to wonder who the hell keeps it going? Not women. A 1992 study conducted for *Sex in America: The Definitive Study,* by Michael, Gagnon, Lauman, and Kolata (Little, Brown, 1994), cited that only 11 percent of females interviewed had purchased X-rated movies and a meager 4 percent had visited a club with nude or seminude dancers in the past twelve months. Compare that to 23 percent of the men interviewed who had purchased an X-rated movie and 22 percent who had visited a "nudie club." Critics in the sex industry said those figures were way too low; they suggested that the men and women surveyed with their spouses present didn't really 'fess up. Even so, that's almost one quarter of the male population partaking in porn! The authors of the study said the patrons of porn movies and strip shows are essentially average people who like sexual diversity. "They are people who are most interested in sex and who find a range of sexual practices very appealing."

You'd be suprised how many guys in suits and men of power prefer—or long for—the realm of the taboo. It goes back to the archetype of Adam and Eve...the forbidden fruit, offered to man by woman. Man wants to taste it and he is willing to pay for the privilege.

Sexual enticement, excitement, and expression is here to stay, and a man needs to experience this part of himself without being considered a pervert or a pig. A man needs a safe place in which to revel in the charms of a female and the scent of a woman. He doesn't always get that in the bedroom, or the boardroom, but he can find it at Scores, a sports bar and strip-club bar in Manhattan, and other places like it around the planet.

"In those places men can be themselves," explains sex therapist Richard A. Cohn, director of the S.I.R.E.N. (Sexuality, Intimacy, and Relationship Enrichment Network) Counseling Center in Los Angeles. "The women who work there get the real thing. At home, the wife gets the homogenized husband who may rein in his sexuality for fear he'll be criticized. A sex worker, or a woman who is so in touch with her sexuality that she can be on the same level with a man, creates a safe place for a man, a place where he can be himself."

Typically a man falls in love—even if temporarily—with one who allows him to express himself this way. That may not be his wife, or the person he stays with, but *it could be*. And many women believe that, in a perfect world *it should be*.

Women Initiating Men

Back to the power of the seductress. Heterosexual men still rely on women to initiate, enlighten, and educate them about sexuality. A woman is also a male's access point for pleasure. While it may sound sleazy, it's not. It's simply nature. Although masturbation is as much a part of *his*-story as intercourse, in order for a man to be truly initiated, he must be accepted and taken in by the female. In our male culture, a man does not become a man until he's had his first woman.

The most legendary tales of men surrendering their virginity in exchange for virility are those that involve an older, more mature, or possibly "professional" seductress who initiated and validated the man through intercourse and *amore*. While young men may

The Seductress and the Sperm

Biology points to the power of the female in inviting and selecting the male. It was long believed by the medical culture that the male played the primary role in conception and that pregnancy occurred only when one mighty sperm made the journey to meet the egg and penetrate its surface.

Over time, scientists and sexologists agreed that the female orgasm in fact is designed to help draw sperm toward its mark. Those delicious contractions of the uterus act as nature's gentle pull of the womb to help suck the sperm upward. This makes a great argument for female pleasure and sexual satisfaction: a women is not only desirous and worthy of pleasure, but *getting it good* means she's doing her job! Female pleasure is nature's way of helping to perpetuate the species.

But wait, there's more. The mighty sperm was king until the very recent discovery that pregnancy is not only encouraged by the female pleasure response, it's biologically determined by the female. The new thinking is that "sperm are ineffectual swimmers," *Newsweek* reported ("The Science Wars," April 27, 1997). "The egg actively grabs the sperm, and genetic material in the egg alone guides development in the first few hours after fertilization."

This biological discovery is yet another nod to the power of the seductress because what the seductress does is choose the man, attract him to her, and keep him near. In the natural dance of sexuality (not the social and criminal anomalies of abuse and rape, obviously), a woman essentially chooses whether or not to let a man court her, mount her, or even impregnate her, and therein dwells a tremendous power!

brag about taking a girl's virginity, men who are initiated by women are more likely to honor and appreciate female sexuality.

Men who actually learn about love and sex from a woman—as opposed to having to figure it out with a woman—often know more about what pleases a woman. The good news is: A man can be initiated at any age!

The Power of a Woman

The greatest natural resource a woman has is her femaleness. Women have extraordinary power between their legs, and seductresses throughout history have recognized that and worked it! Yet they have also known that the greater power of seduction is between their ears—the mind conjures the thoughts, sets the scene, the pace, and the plan, and puts the belief system in place.

Men and women have their fantasies, yet women have the historical advantage over men in that department—i.e., men often have to pay for fulfillment of sexual fantasies whereas women almost anyplace can find men who would, at no charge, help them fulfill their sexual needs. Another female power is that she can physically disengage from a seduction when it suits her. Even if she is more turned on than a feline in heat, she can turn a man away at the last moment or halt a sex act in progress. It may not be the healthiest thing to have all that blood rushing to the genitals without release, but a woman, more typically than a man, will not suffer physical or mental anguish.

A man, on the other hand, cannot easily disengage from a seductress. To start, he will find her hard to resist. And once she has him under her spell, he will find it impossible to ignore the signals from his own body. His attraction will be indicated by his physical response, and his physical response will, in moments of passion, take over.

Could Caesar refuse Cleo? Could Samson shake off Delilah? Can any hot-blooded man refuse a female who brings him to the edge of the abyss and tempts him to dive, dive, dive, deep into the well of her love? I don't think so. Do you?

The piece of history that gets lost in the sex spin is that most seductresses do love the men they seduce. And if they do take prisoners, they are prisoners of love and intense passion. Ultimately, it is love—not the sex organs—that bond men and women (with a little help from handcuffs, if you're into that!). The goal of this book is to show you the tricks of the trade and point you toward a sacred relationship built on love, trust, and the best sexual self-expression and sharing you've ever experienced!

2

Getting to Know Your Inner Seductress

Even though we all began practicing our personal style of seduction from the time we were tiny tots on daddy's knee, not all women grew up feeling confident, empowered, or entitled to be a powerful seductress. Because we live in a culture that demands women be sexually attractive and yet judges them for expressing that part of themselves, many of us feel cut off from our true inner seductress. This often sets us up for an experience of longing to tap into our deepest sexual nature, yet fearing what may happen or what people will think if we do.

As erotic filmmaker Candida Royalle of Femme Productions told me long ago, "Most women need permission to express themselves sexually and allow themselves pleasure." It is a permission that only we can give ourselves.

It is often the fear of losing control with newfound sexual expression that stands between a woman and her inner seductress—even if it is something that she wants with all her heart. We wonder, What will happen if I let the wild woman in me loose?

Since many of us feel that sexual expression comes from the dark side of our natures, we judge ourselves harshly for our desires because we often interpret the dark side as bad. Acting on desires that emerge from that part of us, we fear, will make us "bad girls." We're further torn by the occasional urging of a voice from within that suggests being a bad girl might be fun. Even sexually savvy, open, and liberated women might be surprised to find how these undercurrents of collective unconscious thoughts can affect their self-expression—usually in the form of an insidious, hard-to-pinpoint feeling of guilt—especially when they know that expressing the sex goddess within them is all about having permission to be oh so good *and* oh so bad!

Discovering your inner seductress is like tapping into your own spirit. As a result, you will help heal the split in your female nature and will begin to trust your own instincts and inner direction. It will help you own your power as a seductress, rather than utilize it inappropriately to trap men or sabotage yourself. This chapter is designed to help you perform a reality check on how you think, feel, and act as well as inspire and guide you to the next level.

Embracing the Dark and the Light

It's impossible to express our truest sensuality when we are cut off from an essential part of ourselves. Every woman has her own personal history and background to consider, but I believe that at the root of our sexual fear is the wound of the Madonna/whore complex, a cultural attitude as old as time itself. It is a view that holds women to an either/or scenario: You are either a saintly mother or a lowly slut. The truth is that within each of us dwells both the dark and the light side, a Madonna *and* a whore. It is totally acceptable—in fact, preferable—to embrace and express yourself with a wide spectrum of sexual energies.

While interviewing world-renowned healer and author Deepak Chopra, I gained some insights on this. "True spirituality has to do with being genuine and authentic," he said. This holds true for the inner sex goddess as well. In order to be authentic one must accept all elements of oneself. "Be comfortable with the sinner, with the sacred and the profane, all simultaneously," he suggested. "Be comfortable with the poles of opposite that make life what it is. Dark is your hidden self, your shadow self. Be comfortable with it. It's okay, everybody is like that."

While you are exploring ways to bring your inner seductress out to play, it will be normal to try things that seem out of character; you might find that your inner seductress likes to play with a whip or dreams of stripping for one or more men. Even if it seems totally out of character for you, it's important to allow this part of you to emerge without judgment. Observe your thoughts, feelings, and actions, and listen to your dreams, but try not to be critical.

Anyone can learn to strip or give great oral sex. But just imagine getting in touch with your genuine sex goddess, the inner seductress who lives inside your heart and soul; the one who whispers to you, from time to time, and stirs your desire to be more of who you already are; the one who urges you to be true to yourself and be real with a man.

Developing the courage to express more and more of your inner seductress can lead you to discover your true power as a woman. From this vantage point, you can attract the right man to you or transform existing relationships. You can go way beyond the bedroom to a sacred relationship in which you feel honored, adored, and appreciated by a very special man. First, learn to honor your history and your current reality—even if you don't like it—and the process of your own transformation. For me, the process took many years; I had fun along the way, but it took time to trust my inner voice and follow my heart. Expressing my inner seductress exactly as I wanted to was not an overnight achievement, yet each step built naturally on the next.

An Evolutionary Process

The process of becoming the seductress you truly want to be is a slow and gradual learning experience. It's a process of evolution— not a sudden revolution. In order to truly tap into the treasures of the sex goddess within it is essential to develop a sense of who you are now and how you would like to express more of yourself as a seductress. Much of the process is a fact-finding mission: gathering information on many types of seductresses and styles, culling the elements that most suit you, and then slowly testing the waters.

Drastic changes often result in drastic retreats from change. If you try to transform yourself from Martha Stewart to Madonna overnight, your subconscious mind is going to kick up a storm of resistance and drive you to retreat back to where it's comfortable and safe. Take it slow. Start in your comfort zone and move out of it at a comfy pace.

For example, if it has long been your fantasy to be bathed and soaped by your lover, first give yourself the bath of your fantasies, with all the trimmings like candles, scented bath oil, sultry music. Experience it on your own, so you know what it's like and learn what you like about it. Do it more than once; do it as much as possible. Get used to what it is like to have a wonderful, nurturing, sensual bath privately before you introduce the idea to your lover. When you feel you have mastered the experience, show him what most pleases you. You can do this by example— inviting him to bathe—or through instruction by setting up the environment, running the water, taking him by the hand into the bathroom and leading him through the ritual. Ultimately, you can teach him how to please you this way—but first, you must go through the steps of getting comfortable with the idea and learning to please yourself.

If what you want is to enhance your relationship by being more playful and spontaneous with your man, again, practice in a safe space. Is the kitchen your haven? Start with something small: when your guy comes home from work, just loosen his tie and give him a bigger, longer-than-usual welcome home kiss. Maybe next time you'll unbutton his shirt a few buttons and give him a longer kiss. And maybe the next time you'll unbuckle his pants while you put dinner on warm and lead him to the bedroom. Maybe you'll work up to doing it right on the kitchen floor—or on the dining room table!

While those scenarios may seem unlikely for a shy and reserved woman—or for a busy working woman—remember…inside lives a beautiful, resourceful seductress and the tools to become more of the seductress you truly want to be. Awareness will help you bring her out. Practice will change your perspective as it gives you new skills.

It's like learning to play a new instrument. At first, you may believe you could never in a million years master the piano. Then one day, you find yourself pounding on the ivories. You may sound terrible when starting out, but after a while you will focus more on the activity of playing the piano and getting better at it, rather than focusing on how bad you are. A combination of intention, instinct, instruction, and practice makes the impossible quite possible in a reasonable amount of time.

Go at a pace that is comfortable for you, then challenge yourself from time to time to take it another step further. Make every little bit count. The more aware you become of what you already have to offer as a seductress, the more comfortable you will be, the more skills you will acquire, and the closer you will come to living out your fantasies.

What Magnetizes a Man?

A comment made by my hunky dentist recently confirmed my belief that while men are awed by physical beauty, they are magnetized by a woman's natural sensuality and seductiveness. My dentist, a handsome, sexy, fortyish doctor who is the kind of man that women go for—big time—has had a lot of experience with female seduction of all kinds and says that what attracts him most to a woman is the way *she just is* in her own skin.

He agrees that women often make the mistake of believing they have to be a certain way, do a certain thing, or have a certain skill to get a guy's attention. He says, however, that when a woman *tries* to be a seductress she is not; it's a turnoff. "What I am attracted to in a woman is what's there," he says. "It's not something blatant or forced. Someone who is naturally sexual and seductive just exudes it. I think it comes from their presence, not anything in particular they do or say."

When you clear your mind of the mental images of seductresses you are *not,* and begin to let yourself see the seductress you *are,* then seducing a man becomes an expression of who you are—not just a demonstration of something you learned in a book! And when you fully acknowledge your starting point—whether you're clueless about seduction or you're as skilled as a professional sex worker—you can add to your repertoire in a natural way.

The Wild Woman Within

The world is filled with images of sex. We are bombarded daily by blatant advertising and subliminal media messages that plant images of what a seductress is supposed to be. The truth is, most of us will never look like a model or a movie star; the other truth is, *we don't have to.* A woman doesn't have to fit into size-six jeans or a 36C bra in order to fit the bill of red-hot seductress. Sadly, that is perhaps one of the hardest messages to get through to women today because our self-images are consistently assaulted by what California psychiatrist Judith Orloff calls "Madison Avenue psychosis."

"It's so important for women to get beyond the images and distorted visions that are constantly presented to them in advertising and media and get in touch with their own inner sensuality," says Orloff, author of *Second Sight* (Warner Books, 1997). "No matter what age, what size, what background a woman comes from, her sensuality and seductiveness are a primal feminine force that continues on through life."

Orloff believes that an inner seductress lives within every woman and can be called upon at any moment. First, we have to make initial contact, which Orloff suggests doing through an honest assessment of one's behavior and desires. She says:

> I believe truth is very erotic and when a woman tells the truth about who she is and what she wants, it's powerful. Inside there is a well of passion to call upon. Women can train themselves to call upon this deep, primal, raw energy to come through them. It's so seductive because it is honest—it's not them trying to act like someone they think they're supposed to be. It's expressing the archetypal wild woman, which is, to me, the absolute glory of being feminine.
>
> When you are in touch with that aspect of your seductress within, it doesn't matter what you look like, it has more to do with the expression of energy that's flowing through your body. And it's like invoking the spirit of the seductress you choose to be. When you share this energy with a man it is very healing, it is a great gift to him. It is also like a pheromone!

As you begin to make your acquaintance with and embrace the sex goddess who dwells within, your way with men will flow naturally.

The True Power of a Woman

There's a wonderful line delivered in the movie *Bull Durham* by seductive actress Susan Sarandon in the role of Annie Savoy: "Honey," she says to Kevin Costner, who plays Crash Davis, "this world was made for people who aren't blessed with self-awareness." It's true. From the time we are little girls we are encouraged to be like the other girls and follow the trends; the most "individualistic" are the first ones to follow the newest trend.

I think the true power of seduction for a woman is self-awareness. When you truly know yourself and your desires, you can create a personal approach regardless of what others do or say. When you possess self-awareness—as the actress and her character obviously do—you have the ability to make sound choices. To my mind, self-awareness means you are conscious about life. You are aware of how your childhood and the influences of this culture have helped shape you. You are aware of your desires, and your fears, and have made choices about what you want to focus on in life. With self-awareness, you can transform yourself, because you know where you came from, you know where you are in the moment, and you have an idea of where you want to be.

An open mind is the best way to begin the adventure of becoming the seductress you truly want to be. Add a sense of fun, a willingness to experiment, and the understanding that you may change your mind and your style along the way, and you are ready to begin.

Ask yourself: Do you see yourself as a sassy sexpot like Mae West? Could you be comfortable calculating and executing your charms like Cleopatra? Is it your fantasy to be as confident and wicked as a femme fatale? Would you find it extremely satisfying to be a cool, heel-clicking dominatrix? There's no sense in buying a whip when you'd feel far more seductive with a soft, feathery boa! By the same token, if Cat Woman is your favorite seductress, you may not be very happy or at home in the role of demure, unassertive chambermaid.

We all have fantasies and desires we wish we could find the courage to live out. This is your chance to see where you stand on your own personal seduction scale and chart a path for the future!

Your Seductress Starting Point

Know where you are so you can get where you're going: Take a subjective, up-close-and-personal look at your own style of seduction and sexual self-expression. Acknowledge what you like, and think about how you may want to expand your horizons. This is not a test. You can choose more than one answer. The idea here is to use these questions as part of your fact-finding mission— they will give you a sense of your current seductress status.

You consider yourself:
   a. Sexually open
   b. Too uptight and reserved
   c. Willing, ready, and in need of some tips
   d. Confused about seduction
   e. Other

What is your primary way of getting a man's romantic attention? You:
   a. Soothe and allure him with words
   b. Woo and wow him with a certain outfit or look
   c. Invite him, with your eyes, to come closer
   d. Tell him you want him through actions and statements that make your intentions clear
   e. Other

Which approach best sums up your seduction style?
   a. Blatantly sexual and able to come on strong
   b. Coy and indirect

  c. Sly and cunning
  d. Shy and subliminally seductive
  e. Other

Everyone has a fantasy of being able to be like someone else or
having the courage to do something they've always desired but
feared trying. Who would be *your* favorite role model?
  a. A strong, confident woman who knows what she wants
  b. A sexy, alluring vixen who is irresistible to men
  c. A cool, standoffish female who men clamor for
  d. A gal who knows how to be friendly, open, and avail-
     able to men in a way that makes them feel welcome
  e. Other

Which of the following famous females best embodies/expresses
the kind of seductive charm and allure you admire?
  a. Andie McDowall
  b. Marilyn Monroe
  c. Madonna
  d. Sharon Stone
  e. Sandra Bullock
  f. Other

Choose the female character in a movie that most matches your
fantasy of how you wish you could be with men.
  a. Susan Sarandon in *Bull Durham*
  b. Kim Basinger in *9½ Weeks*
  c. Jane Fonda in *Barbarella*
  d. Rita Hayworth in *Gilda*
  e. Vivien Leigh in *Gone With the Wind*
  f. Other

To you, unleashed, uninhibited passion means:
  a. Going to Chippendales and slipping a dollar to a male
     dancer

    b. Sexual surrender in which you lose control—and love it!

    c. Going nuts with your guy and cheering at a hockey game

    d. Talking dirty and saying things that would ordinarily make you blush

    e. Other

When you slip into something sexy it's usually:

    a. His oversized shirt

    b. A silky nightgown or teddy

    c. A bustier and thigh-high stockings

    d. A clean new bra and cotton underwear

    e. Other

In your secret fantasies, you would love to be able to wear, and carry off, something daring, such as a:

    a. Black leather minidress, bustier, and thigh-high boots

    b. Patent leather raincoat with nothing under it

    c. Form fitting, low-cut gown with thigh-high slit and five-inch heels

    d. Scanty, see-through blouse without bra

    e. Other

Your idea of a hot night is:

    a. Making out in front of a fireplace

    b. Going to a sex club

    c. Being alone in a romantic locale with your honey

    d. Dancing to the beat of Caribbean congas by the ocean

    e. Other

Spontaneous sex for you is:

    a. Running off to have a quickie in a motel room that can be rented for three hours

    b. Doing it on top of your desk

   c. Making love while leaning over a balcony or railing if
      the spirit moves you
   d. Simply not refusing the invitation if presented at the
      right time
   e. Other

The last time you seduced a man was:
   a. Last night
   b. Last week
   c. Several months ago
   d. Can't remember
   e. Other

Be a "Conscious Seductress"

Use the above as points to ponder your seductive nature. Do you
think you are playful and happy-go-lucky, or do you find you are
serious and a little uptight? There is no right or wrong way to be,
but assessing where you are is the first step to knowing where you
want to go. The delightful aspect of consciously charting your
current realities and future fantasies is that it puts you in control of
your own destiny. If you know that you want to be Barbarella
(played by Jane Fonda in the sixties, she was a space vixen who wore
super-sexy outfits, naturally exuded a sensuality that never went
unnoticed by men, and loved sex) in the boudoir, you can aspire to
that. And if you discover the Barbarella thing is just a fantasy, not a
lifestyle choice or even something you care to experience once,
then you can focus on engaging in activities that please you.

    Happy women are a terrific turn-on to men! A woman's true
joy, and unbridled self-expression, is one of the hottest
aphrodisiacs on the planet! Playing the seductress, as opposed to
being one, will turn off the guys. Authenticity will go a long way,
and you will find your genuine seductress as you peel away the
layers of your mind the way a belly dancer peels away her veils.

Review Your Personal History

It's always useful to recognize the early life experiences that shaped your evolution as a woman. Knowing where you came from can also help clarify how you operate today. While you cannot turn back the hands of time to change anything that may have occurred, it is within your power to heal old wounds and be done with the past. Sometimes closing the door on one chapter is a way to begin anew. For some people, simply recognizing a behavior that began in childhood is a way to understand any blocks or confusion about seduction today. Other women are shocked when they realize they are carrying out a Seductress M.O. based on an inappropriate or outdated childhood model.

The following questionnaire is not meant to substitute for a therapist, but rather for you to you spell out defining moments in your seductress evolution. Again, this information is for your personal reference only:

Your father is your first date, your first love, and your first role model of male behavior toward women. You learn about sexuality and seduction through observations and experiences with your father or other significant male adults— by seeing how he interacts with your mother, your sisters, his mother, and you. What kind of lessons in love did you learn from your father?

- a. Men love, adore, and cherish their women
- b. Males appreciate the company of women but do not take them seriously as partners
- c. The man of the house is king and the females are his servants
- d. Men can do anything they please to women, including abuse them
- e. Other

Your mother is your first teacher of how to be a seductress and you often learn a bevy of tricks from her, although you do not recognize them as a child. Some children develop patterns similar to those of a parent and some go in the opposite direction. What kind of role model for sexuality and seduction was your mom?

    a. A sexy vixen who always looked pretty and wanted to please Dad

    b. A working mom who ran the household, her job, your life, and tried to keep up with Dad's needs

    c. An independent, fiery female who felt it was the man's job to come to her

    d. A mild-mannered, demure housewife who didn't speak up or demonstrate enough for you to learn from

    e. Other

When you think back on your parents' relationship, what image of couplehood most comes to mind?

    a. Ward and June Cleaver (in *Leave It to Beaver*)

    b. Blake and Crystal Carrington (in *Dynasty*)

    c. Ralph and Alice Kramden (in *The Honeymooners*)

    d. Archie and Edith Bunker (in *All in the Family*)

    e. Stanley and Stella Kowalski (in *A Streetcar Named Desire*)

    f. Rhett Butler and Scarlett O'Hara (in *Gone With the Wind*)

    g. Tim and Jill Taylor (in *Home Improvement*)

    h. Spencer Tracey and Katherine Hepburn

    i. Richard Burton and Elizabeth Taylor

Try to remember things you overheard or were told about women and sexuality during your formative years and see if any of the following sounds familiar:

    a. Sex before marriage is wrong

b. Girls who express their sexuality around guys are loose women
c. A man will never respect you if you put out
d. A man will never stay with you if you don't put out
e. Women who wear sexy clothes are looking for trouble

Which of the above do you still believe? Why?

Where did you learn the most about sexuality and the nature of seduction?
a. Movies, television, or books
b. School
c. Friends
d. Mom, older sisters, or aunts
e. Religious leaders or doctors

Did any of those influences leave a lingering message? Can you put it into words?

Write a brief description about losing your virginity. Include your age at the time, your relationship with the man, whether it was positive or negative, and what you felt about your partner and yourself at the time.

For example: I was fifteen and he was seventeen. He was my first real sweetheart. I was totally in love but scared. I wasn't really ready but I felt it was inevitable. I believed he was in control. I had no idea what would happen, or how it would feel; I didn't even know his penis had to be erect because I'd never seen one before. I felt inexperienced yet initiated; I felt that surrendering my hymen was like losing an impediment to pleasure. It was a beautiful first relationship. We learned about sex together and it helped me have a positive attitude about sex.

If you could change anything about your first time, what would it be?

    Examples: fear and lack of education, the locale, the guy, etc.

Today, how do you express your sensual, seductive self?
    a. Cautiously
    b. Only with the right person
    c. With all the lights out
    d. With a sense of adventure
    e. With great pleasure

How would you like to express your sensual, seductive self?
    a. Freely, with a sense of ease
    b. Respectfully, with proper reserve
    c. Gracefully
    d. With discrimination
    e. With great pleasure

Can you come up with at least one statement that, without judgment, states how your early influences may have set the tone for how you express yourself today?

Now write at least one statement that summarizes how you would like to express yourself as a seductress. This can be something totally new or something you've known for some time.

Seductress Summary

Your answers to this questionnaire are designed to get you thinking. This seductress summary is designed to get you moving forward on your journey to discovering your inner seductress! Based on the information you've gathered, write down responses (if applicable) to the following statements. Put each response on a separate sheet of paper, the size of an index card.

1. If I grew up with any negative image of a seductress, it was that she is...

_____

Examples: a bad girl, a loose woman, a slut, etc.

2. If I grew up with a negative view of females expressing their sexuality, it was because...

_____

Examples: it's not ladylike, not appropriate to be sexual, etc.

3. If I had to describe the kind of seductress I can see myself becoming, it's...

_____

Examples: a fearless flirt, a man magnet, someone not afraid to show some cleavage, a cool, calm, and collected sex vixen, Madonna, etc.

Exercise

As a symbolic gesture that you are ready to let go of outdated beliefs that get in the way of your sensual self-expression, take the pieces of paper upon which you responded to statements one and two and prepare to discard them in one of the following ways:

Burn them in your fireplace.
Bury them in your backyard.
Tear them into tiny pieces and flush them down the toilet.

Although this would be considered a metaphysical approach, the conscious choice to rid yourself of those beliefs will register with your subconscious and begin the process of transformation. The physical action of burning, burying, or flushing (a handy alternative for urban dwellers!) actually sends a message to your subconscious mind that you mean business and clearly desire a change.

Keep the piece of paper that contains the first description of

Beauty Ritual

When you know you will have quiet and private time at home, dim the lights, play your favorite music, strip off all your clothing, and observe yourself in the mirror.

Look at your body without judgment. Notice your curves and your coloring, your breasts, your behind, and all the areas you do not normally look at: armpits, knees, toes, fingertips. If your eyes begin to focus on the parts of you that make your flinch, find another place to focus. The more you can begin to focus on seeing your most beautiful self, the more beautiful you will become, right before your very eyes. Beauty, as they say, is in the eye of the beholder. If you are someone who has disliked your looks, it's time you know that what you have is a distorted image of yourself based on old beliefs about what is beautiful and what is not.

After you have surveyed the skin you are in, let your eyes catch those of the woman in the mirror. See the sparkle in those eyes and then look beyond it. Try to connect with the goddess within you. She is beyond your body, beyond the sparkle, and way beyond the critical beliefs you may have about your looks—and yet, right there. She comes from a place where there is no such thing as flat-chested, fat, or ugly. She is pure and untouched by the world that has tried to make her believe she is not pretty or sexy or busty enough. Look into your own eyes and see if you can find her there.

Do this "beauty ritual" as often as you can. It only takes about fifteen minutes.

your inner seductress; it will serve as a visual mantra. Displaying your new goal will help you focus on registering it as a new belief.

Studies have shown that anything we focus on, visualize, and give our attention to can be made a reality. So take the piece of paper with the response to statement number three and tape it where you will see it many times a day: on your computer, your desk, your bathroom mirror, or the refrigerator. Write in big letters, type it up, or copy it and plaster it around the house. You will find over time that your written words will act as an affirmation of the sex goddess in your soul.

Your ideal seductress may change over time; that's fine. Use your response to statement three of the Seductress Summary as the kickoff point.

Time Brings Change

As you read on you will find that some of your old beliefs about seduction will begin to fade away. That's a good thing because as you let go of old attitudes, new ones can begin to develop. It all signifies progress in tapping into your inner seductress and inviting her into your life!

How will she help you to seduce a man and keep him under your spell? When you focus your natural seductive energies, you harness one of the most potent forces in the universe. Ask any man to verify that!

3

Unleashing the
Sex Goddess

Before you set about seducing a man, you have to further clarify
what turns you on and brings you pleasure. Although man-
pleasing is certainly part of your game plan, you will find it much
more fulfilling and loving if pleasure is a shared experience. To
become the seductress you want to be, you first must tap into your
fantasies and desires. It is the most potent way to unleash the sex
goddess in your soul.

Some fantasies are meant to stay that way—as fantasies that
fuel the imagination in thought, not action. And some are meant
to be lived and experienced fully. The first part of spreading your
wings as a seductress is to see how far you want to fly. It's
important to allow yourself to evoke your own fantasies and
desires without judgment. The erotic thoughts and desires we try
to suppress the most are the ones that most often turn into
obsessions; things that are left unsaid will often fill every moment,

thought, and experience because we are trying so hard not to think about them! The seductress who learns to own her lust, including her kinky side and even her darker surges of sexual desire, is a woman of great power—and a man magnet supreme!

Write Your Own Story

The most effective way I know to clarify goals, express fantasies, and make desires and dreams come true is to put them into words. When you think about it, everything starts with the written or expressed word; writing helps to formulate things, revamp them, and make them real.

Erotic writing is a great way to get your vital juices flowing and begin to chart a seductive plan of action. It helps you to clarify your true desires, reveal your hidden fantasies, and give language to the pleasure you would like to share with your beloved, or your beloved-to-be.

Putting your passionate pen to page is a way of creating a road map for your journey to becoming more of the woman you choose to be. It is a way of releasing inhibitions, formulating fantasies and fun ideas, creating sensual environments, and developing a penchant for passionate talk. Being able to write the words you always wished you could call out in the heat of passion, and developing the sensual scenes you long for in your current relationship or with a new man you hope to bring into your life, is a way to expand your comfort zone.

Every woman has her own method for crossing the line from feeling she absolutely cannot do something to suddenly (or eventually) feeling that it has always been a part of her life. For me, dirty words were a vexing problem. As much as I longed to use four-letter descriptions of sex-flesh, particularly in bed, I was petrified that it would sound stupid or vulgar.

In the 1980s, I broke through my own inhibitions about descriptions of human anatomy that made me blush by dating a porn editor who was an amazingly sensitive, sweet, and kind man—in addition to being an adventurous Scorpio lover. He encouraged me to write from below the belt. We remained friends, and years after the affair he gave me my first X-rated assignments: two stories on hot love between older women and younger studs, for which I was paid a whopping fifty dollars.

I sweated over those stories as I would a news feature, yet I clearly remember the extraordinary feeling of freedom, release, and renewal I had after pulling the final version from the typewriter: it was pure bliss. In fact, it was better than sex! I felt free, unencumbered, and alive with sizzling passion.

That evening I was at a party filled with the kind of men I ordinarily felt I had to work hard to impress. However, those men swarmed around me. I didn't look or act different, but I was changed. I was the Princess of Passion. It was like the night I lost my virginity—I felt like a total woman for the first time. Having successfully completed two erotic stories, I felt initiated! I had used a lot of "dirty words," written about taboo topics, been the baddest girl I could possibly be, and my entire being brimmed with delight.

That evening a man I'd had my eye on for some time came up and said, "Can I talk to you privately for a moment?" I walked with him to a secluded area in the huge nightclub. He simply looked me in the eyes as if I were the most irresistible woman he'd ever seen and gently kissed me. With just the right touch of take-charge male energy, he walked me backward, gently pressed me against the wall, and smooched as if he really meant it.

Interestingly, it was almost exactly like the scene I had completed writing that day, where the sexually savvy female exudes an irresistible charm that subliminally seduces a man to fulfill her fantasy—without ever having to say anything. It was my fantasy of the moment to be taken, seized, and kissed by a man who really meant it—and the man who was kissing me was someone I desired! That scene with a man who would go on to become one of my significant lovers, was one of many that would prove to be fantasies come true as a result of giving language to my desires by writing them down as lists, in letters, and eventually in published books.

An Erotic Wakeup Call

Erotic writing woke me up. It made me come alive with pleasure and feel that all of life was one big ongoing date. It also whetted my appetite for uncensored writing, and in 1990 I found my niche, starting as a freelance sex editor who added steamy, and steamier, scenes to existing novels, and then as an author. It was the most liberating writing I have ever done—because I could go out and research it personally, or just make it up! I had permission to unleash my sensual self in the most delightfully decadent ways.

Melanie Votaw, a singer and songwriter who pens erotic poetry and teaches how-to courses at the Learning Annex in New York, says that expressing herself in that way is a poetic license that gives her erotic license. "It's a way to own your fantasies and make them come true," she says.

When you give language to your sexual desires you are taking charge of sexual situations. You can become the ultimate seductress, the one you always wished you could be, by living vicariously through characters of your own creation. Or you can choose to experience firsthand the stories you write by turning them into personal screenplays that star you and your beloved.

In either case, writing is a wonderful method of clarifying and concocting. It gives you the chance to see which fantasies you truly lust after and want to experience, and which are merely meant to remain that way—fantasies!

Erotic filmmaker Candida Royalle told me she gauges the sexual potency of her work by how it makes her feel. "If I get turned on by a scene I write or direct, I know I am doing my job," she says. "And I know my viewers are going to get turned on."

Any woman can use erotic writing—in any form—to turn herself on. If you feel aroused while writing your personal seduction scene, it is a sure sign that you are on the right track of expressing your desires. Your state of excitement will also translate to your man—or men—whose attention you are trying to get.

Erotica From a Woman's Perspective

The concept of erotica from a woman's perspective is not just a masturbation tool or a replacement for sex-in-the-flesh (which, let's face it, it sometimes is) but a vehicle through which women can evolve sexually as readers and writers. It's a way to design your experience. If you put your passions on paper and give life to your seductive abilities in words, you then have a blueprint for personal experience.

For example, before a date or a night alone with the hubby, you can write a brief scenario of your vision for the evening. It might go something like this:

The Scene The apartment is filled with beautiful candles of all shapes and sizes, making the place glow with sexy lighting. The energy in the room feels sensual and is filled with possibilities. Anticipation pervades the room. The scent of jasmine (or lavender, fresh strawberry, favorite perfume, whatever) fills the air. Each breath I take brings me great pleasure.

The Experience When he arrives at my door, I am naked beneath a flowing, silk, see-through robe. His eyes connect with mine and he drinks me in with his gaze. Just his being there turns me on and I know it is the same for him. We fall into one another's arms and begin dancing to the sensual tune that plays in the background.

The Feelings I feel so in love and alive that I am irresistible and beautiful. My being brims with passion and desire to experience him with every cell in my body. He knows I want him.

I feel brave and open enough to let him know how important he is to me. I let him know how turned on I am and how good I feel, because I know that will draw him in closer, give him great comfort, and allow him to open to me.

The Aim Tonight we can create the space to open to one another, and go deeper in our love than ever before. I want to feel him filling me, all of me, with love. I want to take him deeply inside, not just physically, but spiritually. I am ready for us to become one.

The Moment You're Waiting For I am ready to practice the esoteric sex secrets I've been studying on the sexy videotape that shows couples engaged in Tantric sex. I've longed for this special moment with him tonight, to climb atop him and allow him to penetrate without moving, and just give himself to me as I give myself to him. First, I want to experience the great pleasures of his tongue and fingers, and then give to him the same sensual joys. I want to feel my entire being filled with joy and make it last—or at least open the doorway to doing this together again.

Of course, it is also perfectly fine if your fantasy scene is about you dominating him, or him just serving you with pleasure all night. Whatever you want can be yours, without judgment. Setting the scene in writing is just one way to bring yourself, and your partner, closer to actually sharing the experience of your dreams.

Let Him Play Too!

Over time, as your confidence builds, you may want to share your fantasy scenarios with your lover. A good way to get what you want is to let him read what you've written—however crude or lewd it may be. Men have a tendency to turn on to a woman's erotic writing. If he knows he is the star, he will probably be more than happy to have a look!

When you really get comfortable with erotic writing, you might find the ritual of writing together is one of the most stimulating and fun activities you can do together—short of living out the scenes with each other. When you can write sexy stuff with a man it brings you closer, and you can learn more about what turns him on and see if it would turn you on to fulfill his fantasy.

Sometimes it feels more natural to write about the two of you, in first person; and some people might find it easier to use made up characters with different names. The beauty is that you have permission to live vicariously, and create vicariously, through your characters. So when you write about those characters, make sure you include all the magic of seduction you want to experience. In fact, you can use some of the insights gained in the last chapter to outline your vision of your inner seductress—the sex goddess of your soul. Ask yourself: *Who is she? What is she like? How does she express herself? What is the look in her eye?*

Enhancing Your Sex Goddess

You might find it helpful to begin a checklist of the kind of seductress qualities you have and those you want to express more. One list can contain an acknowledgment of what seductive qualities you already know and like about yourself; another can be a wish list of qualities you want to enhance and develop.

For example, the first list might read:

I have sensual eyes; I know how to give a man that come-hither look; I'm comfortable with my own sensuality; I like men and their sexuality; I have fun talking about sexual things with guys; men are turned on by my openness.

The other list might contain something like this:

I want to be cool and confident; I'd like to wear low-cut blouses and big-rimmed hats like a classic femme fatale; I'd like to love being in my own skin; I'd like to be able to wear stiletto heels from time to time; I want to say the sexiest things.

After the two lists of seductress "I am's" and "I wanna be's" make a list of fantasies you would live out if you had all the qualities on your wish list in place:

I'd love to be as daring and bold as Cleopatra where men are concerned; I wish I could play dominatrix for just one night; I'd like to get a nurse uniform and ask my boyfriend to play doctor with stethoscope, speculum, latex gloves, and all; I'd like to strip for him on the roof, beneath the moonlight; I'd like to wear crotchless pantyhose and put his hand between my legs during dinner; I'd like to say whatever comes to mind when we make love, no matter how "dirty" it sounds!

Then try this assignment: Pick one seductress quality to try on for size and just do it. Maybe it just means buying a new a low-cut shirt and a Wonderbra (one of those sexy, satiny underthings that push your breasts up higher than they've ever been before) and wearing them in public. Just pick one thing that will help you build toward your goal; trying it will be a declaration that you are consciously evolving into the seductress you choose to be.

Next, pick one fantasy you'd like to live out and try it. You can warm up by writing it down in a story or screenplay, or sitting around and daydreaming; or you can practice on your own for the big moment. Get a whip, stand in front of the mirror and say four-letter words out loud or practice groaning and talking dirty.

It may seem goofy, but it's your first step to achieving the goal. If you are the kind of person who can jump in once you've clarified your desires, then by all means do it. But if you're a little shy, at a loss for words, or new at this, you might want to take it slow.

Know What You Don't *Want*

Erotic writing is a way to learn what you do want; erotic reading is often a way to get ideas, and also learn what you don't want! As you evolve the sex goddess within and bring her out to play more often, it is important that you recognize and accept the things you don't want to experience or even get next to. This will, in the long run, steer you clear from getting involved with men who have seduction fantasies that are not matched with yours.

Make a list of the kinds of sexual expression, encounters, and fantasies you clearly want nothing to do with. It can include anything you feel really strongly about: sex including anyone in addition to you and your lover; experiences with negative or toxic people; S&M; mushy love talk; young guys; old men; women; etc. Take that list and dispose of it the way you ditched some of the beliefs you disposed of in the last chapter: burn it in your fireplace, bury it in the backyard, tear it into tiny pieces and flush it down the toilet.

You are fully entitled to not engage in anything that is not within your comfort level; and, just as important, not to get involved with seductive experiences that do not feel right for you personally. Follow your heart, and you will be guided by the seductress within!

Expanding Your Comfort Level

On the other hand, if your "not" list has anything on it that you would secretly love to experience but which scares you, double-check to see if fear is stopping you from having what you want.

I've written my way through broken hearts and horny nights, and, yes, I've been able to write about the relationships I wish I'd had with the guys who turned out to be so disappointing. I've also used this form of writing to project the kind of experiences I would like to have, and I've rarely been shy about having men read what I've written. In fact, there was a time when reading one of my books was a prerequisite to a date with me.

But it took a long time to get to that place of openness. Most women who place their pulsating pen to page to share or invent a playful erotic tale are not born with said pen in hand. Most of us come to our own eroticism with certain fears of being revealed or judged, and we sometimes need to summon our courage to release all our pent up lust in print. The wonderful, delightful thing about writing is that it gives us permission to come out and play, to say we are sexual beings, to see a cute guy with a great butt and act like a cavewoman in heat—and then write about it! And to use said writing to create a scene, a vignette, or a screenplay about how seduction of or with said cute guy might occur!

If you feel that writing erotically means you have a dirty mind, think again. The experience of writing such stimulating material can often be a catharsis, a clearing, a clean feeling. In fact, one of the perks of being able to write erotic stories is that you may even become a more sincere and direct person. You may find it helps you outgrow some of the agendas you have with men because you will become more directly connected to your own passion and sexuality—and you won't have to rely on the man to help you get in touch with it.

Once you have drawn out your inner seductress you will find that the true powers of a woman are quite magical and awesome, especially when shared with the appropriate guy.

8 Tips on How to Bring Out Your Inner Seductress

1. *Make a declaration.* Accept and appreciate your sexual self-expression as it is today and as it has been in the past, and make a choice about your new direction. Look back at "response three" from the prior chapter—what kind of seductress do you see yourself becoming? When you have more information on the kind

of seductress you would like to be, add it. Reword your statement to say: I have decided to discover my inner sex goddess and become a seductress who....

2. *Ring out the old.* Toss out anything in life that doesn't serve your new goals; let go of things that stand in the way of the wonderful new self-image that will begin to evolve as you become an even more self-aware seductress. Rummage through closets and drawers and discard all of that old stuff: ripped underwear, old bras, pantyhose with runs, clothes that no longer suit you, and anything else that no longer serves you. For this project, use a thirty-gallon garbage bag. Ask yourself: Would a sex goddess wear that getup? Would a sizzling seductress be caught in that old thing? If the answer is no, toss it (or give it away to the homeless or charity).

3. *Create a shrine to the seductress.* Start looking around for little symbols of sexuality and self-expression that represent your new choices, your fantasies, and the fulfillment of desires. These can be statuettes or cute little items like garters or sexual knickknacks that represent your inner seductress. To focus on the sacred, consider a statuette of Aphrodite, the Greek goddess of love, or Oshun, the Yoruba River Goddess of love, beauty, and flirtation, who might each represent a facet of your inner goddess.

4. *Create a visual mantra.* Find one image—preferably a photo of yourself as goddess, but if not then a work of art, a picture from a magazine or a greeting card, or a photo of someone else, that represents the inner beauty you know is within you. Frame it and add it to your altar. It will give you a visual reference for accessing your inner sex goddess. Like a mantra—a symbol that helps you focus on your higher self—it can be a cue that helps you get and stay in touch with your inner seductress.

5. *Make a poster.* Even though I don't want you to buy into the kind of media images that have helped create an epidemic of poor self-esteem in this country, I do want you to utilize any images

that inspire you. Cut out sexy, soulful, colorful images of sensual women, as well as women and men together, from your favorite magazines, and create a poster on a big piece of poster board. Be creative, have fun, go to town with it. The idea is to come up with a collage that represents where you want to go. It can contain images that represent your fantasies and desires, as well as how you would like to look, feel, and express yourself with a man. For example, in my early days of erotic evolution, I cut out an ad of a woman dancing on a tabletop with two men watching and enjoying her state of blissful abandon. She was expressing herself fully. The ad read "No Reservations." It became my theme for becoming uninhibited and free. You will be inspired just cutting out the artwork and magazine photos. As you achieve the goals pictured, you can make new posters.

6. *Use language*. Make sure you cut out headlines and fragments of headlines that summarize your new choices: Sexiest Woman on Earth, Confidence Makes a Woman Sexy, The Woman Men Love to Love, whatever. You can add these to the visual poster or create a word poster that expresses your personal theme.

7. *Learn from movies*. I have learned some of my best moves from movies. I am almost always the only one in the theater taking notes: about how Kathleen Turner stood there trembling with erotic energy in *Body Heat* and let William Hurt hurl a chair through her window to claim her; and how Susan Sarandon tied Tim Robbins to the bedpost and read him literature in *Bull Durham;* how Sharon Stone stared down those cops like an ultraconfident seductress in the famous uncrossing-of-the-legs scene in *Basic Instinct*. Movies are fun to watch, and they can really serve as fodder for the real thing. Take what you like and leave the rest. When translating a film scene to a fantasy, it's appropriate to do some internal film editing.

8. *Say good-bye to Mr. Wrong*. One of the most important factors in seducing a man is making sure that you cast your

seductress spell on the right one. It's possible that you can make a bad marriage good again by bringing yourself more fully to a relationship, and it is possible to pep up a sleepy love life. But don't test your seductions skills on men who cannot, won't, and never will honor you as the sex goddess you are. You know who they are! Think about it the same way you think about that old cotton underwear in your drawer: is he serving me or am I just endlessly serving him? If you are in an iffy relationship now, you will find, over time, that the more you develop respect for yourself, the more respect will shoot right back at you from a romantic partner—or it will send him running. When you learn to let your inner sex goddess lead, she will take you to all the best places!

4

The Modern Seductress and Her Men

Now that you've begun your journey of meeting and becoming your inner seductress, I urge you to stay on the path of self-discovery as you incorporate new aspects of seduction into your self-expression. It's important that you ground yourself in self-awareness and make very clear choices about the kind of man, or men, you want in your world. Why? Because once you start letting the sex goddess in you shine, men will flock around you like lions during mating season.

I kid you not when I say it could start raining men—even if you are already married—because a woman in touch with her sensuality is irresistible to men. Use common sense and intuition to help you pick and choose wisely. Just as in the dating game, not every man who will be drawn to you is appropriate. It's important to stay on top of the seduction, so that you don't fall under the spell of the wrong man.

Men Are Easy

As the Devil says to his star seductress in *Damn Yankees:* "This is a straight seduction job, Lola."

Let's look at the basic tenet of seducing a man: Almost any man—even the great ones, the gorgeous ones, the rich ones, and the ones every other woman covets—is seducible. It is the natural order of things.

If you have even a shadow of a doubt about your powers as a seductress, or feel the least bit insecure about your ability to seduce a man, think again. When it comes to being more easily enticed, or aroused by the presence, energy, or physical being of the opposite sex, men win hands down—and penises up!

I once asked the famous Mayflower Madam, Sidney Biddles Barrow, why there were no rent-a-stud escort services for single, straight women—services staffed by heterosexual hunks who could satisfy a female at whim! "It wouldn't be profitable," she said. "Women don't have to pay for it. Men give it away so easily."

When the chemistry and moment are right, most men are very susceptible to even the subtlest charms of a woman. Not only have we seen it historically, we see it daily in the newspapers and on the six o'clock news. The President of the United States and other prominent men regularly make headlines with alleged sex scandals.

As author John Gray, of *Men Are From Mars, Women Are From Venus* fame, puts: "They set him up with temptation. Unlike women, men get turned on physically first, and then think later."

The modern seductress should never forget that the very nature of the female makes her irresistible to men, and in many cases all she has to do is be in the glow of her own femaleness to attract a man's attention.

Using Your Power Wisely

Obviously, the more in touch with your seductive powers you become, the more you will yearn to demonstrate and share them. It is a natural progression to get excited and horny. But since you are unleashing a power that is irresistible to men, you want to make doubly sure you stay away from those Mr. Wrongs. I know from personal experience that utilizing seductive charms without appropriate discretion or even consciousness can seal a relationship with the wrong guy! I'll share my most potent example.

While working at *Playgirl* I was also working on getting to know my inner seductress. The environment I was in placed great emphasis on celebrities, and one of the first issues I worked on was the "Ten Sexiest Rockers." Rockers had never interested me, yet something came over me: I wanted to date a rocker. In no time, he appeared. Just because he had long hair, wore leather pants, and talked rocker talk (such as, "Oh baby, I love you"; "Oh baby, I wrote this song for you") I unleashed my Seductress Supreme and made myself irresistible on all levels—sexually, socially, and professionally.

He wasn't even a rock star. In the end, I realized I had seduced a fantasy, and had no clue who this guy really was. Why didn't I see it up front? Because I was not coming from my inner seductress, I was coming from the part of me that felt I had to seduce a man in order to get him to like me. At that point in my life, I really didn't know how to let my sex goddess guide me. When you operate that way you are more likely to attract men who are also "performing," or coming from a false or inauthentic part of their personality. When I gave away my power, it was easy for him to keep me as emotional hostage—until I broke free. Even though I got out of the relationship relatively fast, it was months before it was truly over. I had seduced him well! He didn't want to let go. That's when I realized how powerful our female prowess is and how important it is that we use it consciously.

When a man is under your spell, he will stay there for a long, long time, so you want to make sure he can also give you what you need in a relationship. If you slip up, just send him away with your blessing and move on as soon as you can.

Self-awareness and respect for others will go a long way to ensure that you are a seductress of integrity, honesty, and appropriate behavior. Rule out any men whom you really can't have: other people's husbands or boyfriends, priests, and the president of the United States. Then eliminate the ones you really don't want: your boss (or any guy who signs your paycheck), the guy in the office who wouldn't let you live it down, bad boys, abusive men, users, Peter Pans, and anyone who can't eventually engage in the kind of relationship you aspire to.

To make sure you have a vision and a goal for the kind of man you want to meet, make a list entitled "Qualities I Choose in a Man." Even if you don't know who the man is yet, or if you think it's impossible that your husband or boyfriend could ever fit the bill, make the list. This is just another tool to help clarify the type of man who would be your best match; often, just the act of writing it helps you focus your intentions and attentions on appropriate men.

. Some women already in relationships find that when they clarify what they want from their mates, they begin to communicate more openly and effectively with their lovers; it can restore hope to a relationship. As you continue to gather information—through real life experience and personal fantasies you begin to discover—the list may grow and change. But it is a great way to start focusing on whom you will share your delicious sex goddess self with.

Seduction for the sake of sex is fine for consenting adults, but try not to reel in a guy just to use him—even if you are tempted to take some of your new skills for a test drive! While some women are more prone to seducing for their own pleasure, it's always a good idea to play with someone who can handle you and to stay away from people who can be hurt (or who can hurt you!). I call it the "Three Vs Rule" and it should be applied to seduction at all times: Don't seduce anyone who is vulnerable, vindictive, or violent.

Some women develop faster sexually than emotionally in relationships and can utilize sex as a doorway to love. In the process, it is possible to learn about expressing the seductress within in an emotionally safe way. Oftentimes it is easier to practice and master the skills of seduction with men whom you are not seriously in love with. There is less at stake and you won't be hindered by the fear of losing the man or scaring him off! It's not a recommended practice if you are otherwise engaged, but single women should have the same flexibility and opportunities as bachelors!

Sex Rules for Seductresses

Remember this: The sexual genetics set forth by nature, and a collective male unconscious that has for eons evolved a male worldview predominantly from within the general vicinity of a codpiece, has consistently led the male of the species to fall into a predictable pattern. It all boils down to one basic premise: The penis is king. History has shown us that a woman who understands this—or simply activates it—can achieve goddesslike stature in the eyes of men.

How much have modern guys really evolved from their primordial cave brothers? Not much. When you understand that men, in general, follow a certain sexual protocol, you can master the Sex Rules.

1. Every man is seducible and, in fact, wants to be seduced. History has shown us time and again that femmes fatales, sensual

sorceresses, sexy sirens, and hard-to-get women rule because they understand the anatomy of seduction, which is, simply, to understand that men are slaves to their willies, and sex is the universal language of penis owners. You can always get a guy's attention with sex. Men cannot keep from responding to even the subtlest whiff of female sexuality. Even when a guy knows a woman is trouble, or will get him into trouble, he often feels as if he has no control over his reaction. Even if he doesn't respond sexually, he'll respond subliminally.

2. Men want breasts in their faces. From rockers to rednecks, cleavage works. Just as a nursing baby sees a breast and thinks "Dinner!" a man sees a breast and thinks "Dessert!" From the day they're born, almost all males believe breasts are designed for their dining pleasure. Any exposed breast—big or small—is of interest to a male. Mammaries have magnetic powers—the more accessible, the stronger the pull. While it's true that some men are "leg men" or "butt guys," very few heterosexual guys can resist the allure of naked, seminaked, or sort-of-showing breast. A woman's cleavage is another place where men tend to feel a little out of control.

3. The average man wants to express himself…naked. Most men communicate more effectively with women when they are nude. It just seems to work better that way. Men, being creatures of action, are often more adept at running a tongue along all the right places than using that same organ to communicate verbally. But even the most uptight suit can loosen up once his tie is on the floor and he's out of his "armor." He's like a free little boy again when he can get naked and comfortable with you. He's also relieved because he feels his part in the seduction is over and triumphant—he's done the work he was supposed to do if he can get naked with or around you. By the time a guy gets his trousers off, he knows he's going to get sex, so he's relaxed and can demonstrate how he feels by receiving, and giving, pleasure.

4. When a man is attracted to a woman, he imagines what she looks like naked from the moment he first sees her and wants the first hint of sexual suggestion to be his cue to remove all of her clothes. This is one of the toughest rules for most women to negotiate because we like our coverups, props, boob lifts, and tummy flatteners. Some women spend *days* shopping, preparing, and dressing for a sex date and put hours into getting that perfect seductress look (the one where your makeup is *just so,* your cleavage is just right in that fabulous bustier, and your tummy is looking flatter in your new slimmer slip). Although men love it— it gets them hot, lures them in, makes them want you even more—the first thing a guy really wants to do is to shed you of your sin-hiding, sensual fashion statement, wiggle you out of your Wonderbra and sexy garters, and see the goods. Refrain from screaming, *"Hell-o!* Can I keep my clothes on for more than fifteen minutes into the date?"* Although you must learn to tease and tantalize before you get fully naked, he will almost always be wanting you *more naked,* and *naked faster,* than you had in mind. To a man, naked female flesh is assurance of the pleasures to follow. Clothes are generally an annoying block to intimacy that they must remove in order to reach their goal.

5. A man wants a sexually take-charge woman to know what the hell she is doing. Although some men are far too controlling to let you run the sex show, there are those who will want you to *do it to them* with expertise, finesse, and style—so be prepared. If you propose something even slightly kinky to a man, be ready to lead the way, especially if he is the kind of guy who thinks of himself as "macho." A man who feels he must always appear to know what he's doing is often insecure inside; he may not want to admit he's depending on the confidence and sexual skills of a woman because he himself is clueless. You will learn this in the most humiliating way possible if you decide to try something you've never done before with a macho guy who's never done it either—

because he will head for the hills as soon as he realizes the onus is on him. Guys like that would rather hire a pro than chance fumbling around with someone who doesn't know the terrain any better than he does! If you want to venture into unknown territory, do your homework—you can hire the pro, even if it is just to gather how-to tips!

6. Men want erotic clarity. There's nothing like an erection knocking at a guy's belt buckle to make it clear what *he* wants. Guys tend to see things in very black-and-white terms; they get lost in all those gray areas that women live and breathe for. You either want to sleep with him, or you don't; you're either wet down there, or you're not. A man can't relate to the way women "reason" about such things; and a guy is not interested in having a board meeting over whether or not he's going to get any sex. While women can neck and pet, enjoy the contact, and do without the actual act of sex, a man does not fare well with the notion of getting all steamed up and *not* going all the way—unless it is clear from the outset that he is being treated to a delightfully prolonged seduction that will eventually lead to sexual release. Certain actions promise intercourse to a man, so make sure that as a seductress you are communicating the same sex language at the same frequency as your guy.

7. A man *does* want you to get more off your chest than just your bra...but do it *before* he reaches the point of no return. Talking about sex (or anything for that matter) falls on deaf ears once a guy gets that sex-glazed, mad-dog look. Confessions and explanations should take place before he's so turned on that he can't think straight; the moment his manhood is poised at your portal of love is not the time to tell him anything alarming or requiring more than a grunt as acknowledgment. However, men are excellent listeners when they know it will lead to sex. If you let a guy know that you will feel more like a free spirit if you can chat a spell before proceeding to the finish line, most men will want to

hear whatever you have to say. A man who leaves a half-hour grace period in which a woman can "share" considerations, fears, and safe sex issues knows he is a man who is going to get laid, because he makes a gal feel understood. Even seductresses need to be heard by men.

8. All men want to date and mate with a nubile, adoring twenty-one-year-old (preferably model, actress, or dancer). This is a tough one for the seductress who is twenty-two or over, but it's a primal attraction and there's no sense in fighting it. Men have to have their fantasies. They have to be able to look; sometimes, they need to be able to touch. This is what keeps callgirls, strippers, phone sex specialists, and net sex operators in business: At that moment, a man can have his fantasy and maybe eat it too! A guy needs a woman who makes him feel like the king of the world— the most handsome, well-hung, sexy studmeister to grace the earth—at least once in a while. If you want to see how men really respond to being titillated and tantalized by nubile flesh, visit a strip club or a peep show and get a gander at the look on a guy's face. If he can't actually have that nubile twenty-one-year-old, you have to at least let him pretend from time to time. Don't take it personally. You may find it inspires you to play the role sometimes as well. While it may be said that some men are like dogs, you can't put them in the doghouse for following those animal instincts and doing what comes naturally.

9. Men want directions but they don't want to have to ask. They really do want to pleasure women. But if a guy hates stopping at a gas station to figure out where the hell he is, imagine how he'll feel about asking how to find your G spot. Most men want a road map to your pleasure delivered in a way that makes it look like he figured it out himself. Even though he *says* to tell him what you want him to do to you, he'll often only *hear* those directions when it sounds like you're talking dirty. Just preface your preferences with "Oh, baby!" and "Ohhhhs" and" Ahhhhs"

and he will respond. Men have to be naked and in bed, with the opportunity to act out the directive, in order to *really* get it.

10. Men want to feel they've won a prize. Men feel they've won someone special when they have to slay dragons, conquer lands, and move a few mountains to get a woman to say yes! Sensual self expression and sexual assertion are key for a woman's sense of power and self-esteem. It's also important to learn to balance and tread the area between "expressing interest" and seeming "too easy." While men find a female's indecision about sex *(should I or shouldn't I?)* a hideous form of torture, they do love to hunt after a woman who gives good chase. Men are predisposed to want to get into your bloomers; they can also have this nasty habit of thinking you're too available if you let them get there too fast. The ancient game of seduction is still successful in modern times: As long as you give him the sign that he's got a chance, you can tease, tantalize, and seduce him into becoming your devoted love slave—or at least make him your partner in seduction.

Seduction is supposed to be fun and freeing—it's never supposed to be a struggle or chore. If you find yourself struggling in your attempts to discover your inner seductress, try another direction so that you don't get stuck. If you find yourself with a man with whom your attempts to be seductive have become a difficult and draining experience, consider finding a new man. If you know you are with the right person, then take some time to learn a little more about how to communicate and invite him out to play with you.

Always find out what turns him on—make it part of your fact-finding mission as you move forward—but trust that you can seduce a man, keep him under your spell, and enjoy the hell out of it. Once you discover your "Seduction Signature," you're halfway there!

PART II ❤

Learning From the Titans of Temptation

5

You've Got to Have Attitude!

Remember, there are only two things without
limits—femininity and the means to explore it.
—From *La Femme Nikita*

I've had the opportunity to explore many forms of sensual expression—from strip clubs to S&M clubs to Tantric sex workshops. In writing this book I have tried to cull for you some of the most exciting concepts in sensual expression and give you some of the tools with which you can design the environment, mood, and style that will make up your personal "Seduction Signature."

While we can see the success of certain aspects of seduction throughout history, and there are clearly certain types of seductresses that are effective at turning men on, you can't expect to fit into someone else's shoes (or stiletto heels, as the case may be) and act out a role that does not feel right for you. If performing certain acts of seduction makes you gag or feel too vulnerable and uncomfortable, then you know you are not being true to yourself. Try something else!

At the same time, you've got to know the man you are dealing with, even in a new relationship or a potential relationship. You can't take a macho meat-and-potatoes guy who loves football and strip clubs and turn him into a love slave to your dominatrix. By the same token, you can't expect a doctor who needs to be dominated by women to act like a caveman to your Lolita (I know this from firsthand experience). While one man might love to be teased by a femme fatale, another might be able to respond only to a soft and innocent sweetheart or an irresistible sexpot.

This section is like an encyclopedia of information from which you can create your own seduction manual, based on what suits you personally. When you are expressing yourself from the heart, you will know because it will feel good to you, and your man will be wild with passion. If you are tripping over yourself, feeling uncontrollably embarrassed, or not feeling quite right, you may be taking the wrong seduction tack. If you feel good about what you are expressing and your man is not getting turned on, you might simply be with the wrong man! Finding your Seduction Signature style will be a "create and adjust" process!

How the Working Girls Do It

In observing how professional sex workers create allure for male clients, in talking with experts who have studied and trained in various modes of human seduction and sexuality, and having personally jumped into the ring to play a few different seductress roles myself, I've picked up a few key pointers about dealing with men seductively—in both sexual and nonsexual situations.

In the movie *Perfect*, John Travolta confessed to Jamie Lee Curtis that "an interview is like a seduction." As a lifelong journalist, I can relate to that and would add that a good interview is like good sex. To my mind, seduction equals some sort of sexual stirring, satisfaction, or experience, whether consummated or not. These situations are not difficult to come by in life. Working it out so that you, your intended, and your Seduction Signature are, as they say in the publishing world, on the same page, is the challenge. Keep in mind these two points:

1. *Seduction is easy.* I believe that all situations are potential seductions in some sense (whether you're buying a new dress, selling a product, or closing a business deal), and situations that include a heterosexual woman and a heterosexual man in the same place at the same time—crowded subways, the gym, the supermarket, the office—can become sexually charged in nanoseconds. (It's *keeping* a man seduced that is the challenge! More on that later.)

2. *Attitude is everything.* How you put it out there, what you tell the world about yourself with your attitude toward life, is what comes back. How people treat you is a mirror of how you treat yourself. How your man responds to you depends on what you communicate—in words, actions, nuances, body language, eye contact, etc. If you're reading this book because you don't like the response you are getting, or because you want to enhance it, then you might need an attitude adjustment, or a new attitude.

Attitude!

You might already be a woman who is a seductive force to be reckoned with, with plenty of attitude to go around. Don't underestimate your power just because a dominatrix knows how to make men cower and you don't; simply add to your power and enhance your attitude where appropriate by studying some of the "Temptress Traits to Emulate" in the following chapters.

Oftentimes, having role models (famous historical vixens,

movie stars, characters in a film) will help you begin to identify and bring out the right seductress qualities. Sometimes you have to fake it before you make it—so you can learn to get to where you are going.

Acting in ways associated with sexually dominant women or any of your model seductresses could be the first steps to developing and exuding a new attitude. That's why I have tried to outline some of the qualities of seductresses—take those you resonate with and leave the rest.

For example, I could never be a femme fatale, but I would love to be able to pull off the black-hat-and-veil look, and I fantasize about living my life without apologies—two characteristics of the femme fatale. Come to think of it, I wouldn't mind being a sexy siren like Barbarella. Although I am not a Jane Fonda-like beauty, am hardly innocent, and don't even own a car, I can adopt Barbarella's delightfully accepting attitude about feeling pleasure. Just watching the film *Barbarella* raises my energy and puts me in the mood to emulate my favorite roles.

Within all women dwells the desire to be true to our most genuinely seductive nature—a desire to kick all fears out of the way, adopt and adapt some new concepts, and scream (or sing) out, "I got a new attitude!"

Tips for Adapting Temptress Traits

Each of the following chapters has a "Temptress Traits to Emulate" section and a listing of movies that may be useful. The following tips are to help you put some or all of these traits into practice.

Study. Watch films, read books, follow the news on celebrities who have that certain something; notice characters in plays, on TV, in books. There are many sources in which you can find role models, women who have come before you and have mastered a few things you would like to get good at. Keep your eyes open and you will learn a few tricks.

Observe. All of life is fodder for your project of defining your Seduction Signature. It's perfectly acceptable to appreciate the way someone in your office dresses, notice the way a female at a bar throws back her hair, take note at the way your man—or any man—looks at other women. Observation can occur anywhere. Just to get your feet wet, sit in a hotel lobby and people watch for a half hour or more. Notice the people in restaurants and bars. Check out the folks on the street. Seductress tips are in the air, everywhere!

Take field trips. Whenever possible, go to where the action originates and watch the way it goes down. Take a bold female friend who wants to buddy up, or take a guy, and visit a strip club, a sex club, a domination parlor. You? Never? Remember, there's a first time for everything. If checking out a professional stripper is going to give you insights into seduction that will make you feel powerful and knock your lover's socks off, would you let a little thing like being chicken stand in the way?

Seek lessons. Wherever possible, get some training by someone reputable who best expresses the kind of sensuality and energy you would like to express. There are adult education courses and private lessons available in many seduction technologies. If you can't find a course, there are tons of videotapes and books to teach you.

Get coaching. While on my journey of learning my own Seduction Signature, I have taken a prostitute to lunch, spent a day with an erotic filmmaker, interviewed former porn stars, taken dominatrix training and stripping lessons, and have sought insight from many professionals. Sometimes you have to pay them for their time or at least treat them to a meal; often, it is worth it. There is nothing like getting information straight from the source.

Practice. First by yourself, then in the mirror, then with a friend, then with people you don't know, until you break through inhibitions and cross over to the comfort zone.

Dress up and go out. The final frontier for evolving your Seductress Signature is to dress up in full regalia and go out and play. I made my first flesh-revealing fashion statement when I got decked out in my new Barbarella-like plastic, see-through fetish bra and skin-tight black leggings and headed to the Vault, a Manhattan club, with a date in tow. I reveled in the fact that men were looking at me and that a steady stream approached me with one comment or another (even though I had a date with me!). For that moment, I felt like Barbarella—sexy, independent, and free. It was all in my attitude, and the clothing, environment, and attention simply enhanced it.

Work it, Girlfriend. Work that attitude. Get a feel for it, play with it, express it, experience it, see how others respond to it, and work it, wherever you go. The more you work it, the more you become it. The more you express it, the more natural that expression becomes. The more you develop that attitude, the more that attitude becomes a natural part of you. It's a law of the universe!

As my friend Myreah Moore, "The Dating Coach of the 1990s" puts it: "We are all goddesses. And being a goddess is an attitude, something that comes from inside. But, girlfriend, you can help it along with clothes!"

Modern women have a lot to learn from the Titans of Temptation, described in the chapters that follow. These females are the original molds for some of the most exotic, erotic, dazzling, and irresistible seductresses known to mankind! They are the pioneers of seduction, the high priestesses of passion. Although you may not follow the model of any particular seductress, you may find it useful to incorporate snippets from one or more into your life.

6

Lessons From the Femme Fatale

There aren't any hard women, only soft men.
—Raquel Welch in *Hanny Caulder*

The femme fatale is the most infamous and compelling seductress. Although femme fatale is a catch-all label that has been placed on many a passionate woman who owns her power, expresses her sexuality, or has the ability to persuade a man with her womanly ways (it has even been pinned on Mary Magdalene), a real femme fatale is a cold-hearted man killer who mercilessly seduces, uses, and then ditches a guy—usually by getting him to commit a crime on her behalf or at the very least take the fall for it.

Cleopatra and Mata Hari are infamous for using their sexuality to get men to do their bidding—a femme fatale trait. There are witches, noblewomen, and courtesans who followed suit. Some women you read about in real-life justice stories fit the bill, such as the gun moll who manipulated her man into a life of crime (there have been a few) or the teacher who seduced a student in order to get him to kill her hubby. They all have attributes of this type of vixen. But for the most part, a femme fatale is a mostly male invention brought to life in pulp fiction and Hollywood films. She's the ultimate bad girl—a smooth, sexy, countess of cool portrayed by the likes of Bette Davis, Barbara Stanwyck, Joan Crawford, Theresa Russell, Sharon Stone, Madonna.

Perhaps the femme fatale was born out of the fear of female sexual demons—i.e., fear of females and their adept ability to seduce men into doing anything and then ditch them! As the *Encyclopedia of Erotic Wisdom* explains it: "Throughout the world we find a particular female deity of whom it is said that they either seduce or sexually assault men."

This image recalls the behavior of certain females in the animal world, such as the black widow spider, who is known to kill the male after sex, and the even more voracious female preying mantis, whose habit is to bite off the head of her mate during copulation. She starts trying to consume him the moment he gets next to her. But even as she chomps on his head, the part of his body remaining will mount her and copulate. It is said that this is a function of perpetuating the preying mantis species, not just cannibalism, because it's the male's brain that gets in the way of copulation. So she gets rid of it and still uses him until the deed is done.

Sound similar to the femme fatale that men know and love, and can't get enough of, in the movies? It's also reflective of the real male fear of being lost in or devoured by the female's vagina. What's important here to the modern seductress is recognizing that men obviously respond to such a creature. They are repelled and charmed, mystified and horrified, and yet can't help themselves from wanting more. A savvy seductress who finds some of the femme fatale's best features appealing can utilize them in her communication with men.

The Ice Queen

The classic femme fatale is adept at seducing men by being a total ice queen. It proves a point that most high priestesses of passion know about men—if you give a man a whiff of what you've got, it will entice him into seeking out more. When you give him everything, even the most in-love-with-you guy will get bored. The femme fatale has mastered the power of patience. She knows how to keep a guy guessing and yet make him feel like he's getting a piece from a goddess!

The femme fatale exudes a sexual confidence that is intoxicating. Nasty, bitchy, possibly guilty of major crimes (such as murder), she has a sex appeal so hot that, if you can put aside the Hollywood message that femmes fatales are deadly in a literal sense, perhaps it is your most fitting fantasy to be a killer seductress—one who bowls men over with a power they cannot resist. Men break glass (William Hurt, for Kathleen Turner, in *Body Heat*), and have sex on glass (Willem Dafoe, with Madonna, in *Body of Evidence*), just to have a round with a cold-hearted woman who inflames his sexual soul.

My favorite example of a femme fatale supreme is Bridget (the heartless) Gregory, the role portrayed by Linda Fiorentino in *The Last Seduction*. After manipulating her husband-the-doctor into making a drug deal, she steals the money, ditches her marriage, and leaves him at the mercy of a local loanshark. She then finds some cute but pathetic puppy of a guy in a little cowtown called Beston to give her all the sex she wants, kill her husband, and take the fall for it. The grand finale doesn't exactly go as she planned, but that doesn't stop her from getting what she wants. Regardless, she gets away with it. By the end of this movie, you want her to— if only because it proves men are such slaves to their sexual desires that women can get them to do anything!

Fiorentino portrays a woman so cold that her lawyer asks, "Has anyone checked you for a heartbeat lately?" Yet she's a woman so effective that we'd be remiss if we did not acknowledge, and maybe even utilize, some of her tricks.

When local hayseed Peter Berg tries to pick Fiorentino up, she tells him to get lost, until he tosses her a challenge: "I'm hung like a horse. Think about it." Her response is to unzip his pants, feel around "for something of a Mr. Ed–like quality," and quiz him on his sexual history. She then grants him the honor of a sexual affair.

Alas, he asks so many boring, annoying relationship questions that he really gets on her nerves.

"Where do I fit in?" he wants to know.

"You're my designated fuck!" she says.

Clearly, most of us don't want to emulate Bridget's behavior, but in the darkest recesses of the mind there could be a teeny-weeny part of us that would like to—just once—tell a guy how it is and how it's going to be in no uncertain terms. Fiorentino in *The Last Seduction* is an excellent example. This is because she is so exquisitely adept at her personal game of seduction.

While few of us will ever have sex while hanging on a chain-link fence (à la *The Last Seduction*) or kill our mates in cold blood (though we may sometimes fantasize about that too!), there is something to be learned from a woman who does what she wants when she wants and has the brass to use or climb over anyone and anything that gets in her way, and *gets sexual satisfaction along the way.* As long as you don't do anything illegal, immoral, or nasty enough to give you bad karma, why not consider incorporating some of the redeeming qualities of the femme fatale?

Temptress Traits to Emulate

Temptress traits you can safely borrow from the femme fatale, without having to kill anyone, include:

Attitude.   She's got it and knows how to use it. While it's hard to describe exactly what it is, you know it when you see it. She is confident, cocksure, and has no qualms about manipulating the situation. She commands attention. Not only is she a man-magnet, she possesses the ability to pull opportunities toward her. She seduces without apology and exudes a cool and unnerving confidence. She feels entitled!

Wardrobe. She always dresses cool. Wide-brimmed hats with veils, snug and sexy skirts, low-cut necklines—such outfits make a woman feel good in her own sensuality and get a guy's attention. Elegance—in casual, business, and nighttime attire—is key. She wears clothes that push her boobs, and her sexuality, in your face without seeming slutty. While wardrobe is telling on where a femme fatale is at—usually an inflated sense of self-esteem and entitlement—the body also responds to being inside that kind of clothing and assists in sensual expression. Her clothes are usually impeccably classy and sexy. Just developing that look, with elegant suits and short skirts that accent your figure, and accessories that make you feel rich and wicked, is worth the price of movie rentals featuring femmes fatales who dress to kill.

Man-management techniques. The cardinal rule of staying cool and aloof is not to let a man get under your skin. The challenge is overcoming human nature—the desire to be loved—and resisting those pesky guys who just keep on knocking at your door. It's a big problem when a femme fatale supreme succumbs to love; love has brought down some of the brassiest broads in history. Yet civilian seductresses have something to learn from the femme fatale's man-management techniques—she practices self-preservation and gets what she wants. Perhaps there is a way to incorporate those skills into a real relationship?

Mystery. The femme fatale has the ability to create emotional distance (an especially good thing to learn if you're usually on the other end of the spectrum in codependence land), and that makes her bold, daring, and mysterious. A woman who can stir up a little trouble and excitement, who is unpredictable and cannot be possessed, drives a guy crazy and keeps him seduced. The femme fatale opens up the gates of Eden and tempts a man to taste the forbidden fruit. It is a sexual bliss he is more than willing to surrender to; in many ways, he feels as powerless to resist as Adam was with Eve.

Want to Be a Femme Fatale Just for Fun?

Your assignment, should you accept it:

- Watch at least two movies starring femmes fatales you can relate to. Here are some suggestions:

  Greta Garbo in *Mata Hari* (1932)
  Hedy Lamarr in *Samson and Delilah* (1949)
  Elizabeth Taylor in *Cleopatra* (1963)
  Tuesday Weld in *Pretty Poison* (1968)
  Angie Dickinson in *Dressed To Kill* (1980)
  Kathleen Turner in *Body Heat* (1981)
  Theresa Russell in *Black Widow* (1986)
  Annette Bening in *The Grifters* (1990)
  Sharon Stone in *Basic Instinct* (1993)

- Go out and buy or borrow one piece of clothing that is a staple of the femme fatale wardrobe and wear it around the house until you expand your comfort level. Next, dare to wear it out of the house. It might be fun to try on a wide-brimmed femme fatale hat with a black widow veil and dare yourself to wear it out the door. Dressing to kill can take on a new meaning when you slip into something short, snug, and elegant and take on that outta-my-way-buddy attitude that our movie femmes fatales portray so brilliantly!

- Pick a line uttered by your favorite femme fatale and practice saying it out loud when you are alone. Pick a line that sends a chill of excitement and longing down your spine when you first hear it. For example, the classic line uttered by Kathleen Turner in *Body Heat:* "You're stupid. I like that in a man." Make it a part of you. Utter it at least once to someone. Note his reaction. Does uttering these words make you feel more powerful, sexy, or seductive? If so, try it out in real life.

- ♥ Adopt your favorite femme fatale quality—cool, calm, and collected; tough; ice queen—for an hour and try it on for size.

7

Lessons From the Stripper

And when she started to do the Naked Dance
of Love, I knew right then that I was—for a fact—
in love.

—Wayne Rankin, *The Underachievers*

The exotic dancer is a mainstay of the American male culture. In this country, most men know what a titty bar is, and a healthy percentage have actually visited such an establishment at least once in their lifetime. Don't let the pinstripe suits fool you: In metropolitan areas, most of the men who frequent strip clubs seem to be straight and conservative. It is an American male rite to go out with a bunch of buddies and watch a woman dance, strip off her clothes, and wiggle, bump, and grind across a stage.

Exotic dancers come in many forms. There are strippers, who dance, strip off their clothes, and strut their stuff, often collecting dollar bills as they go along; there are table dancers, usually strippers who offer the additional service, at an additional price, of doing private dances for patrons by, or on, the table they're sitting at; and there are lap dancers, women who (naked or scantily clad) mount a man's lap (while he's clothed) and wiggle around in a dry hump, sometimes until he has an orgasm (usually a sport for raunchier clubs).

Some exotic dancers will strip down to nothing, and some leave on a G-string, depending on what kind of establishment and which state you're in. Yet it is not just the seductive promise of naked flesh that makes an exotic dance something men drool over.

What are the secrets of exotic dancers, and how do they get men to fall under their spell? Men adore erotic entertainment and the sight of a sexy siren stripping off her clothes, but one of the most potent powers of a good exotic dancer is her ability to not only dance for a man but to create the illusion of intimacy and passion.

While dancers utilize their flesh, form, and movement to titillate and fulfill a man's fantasy, their most potent weapon is their eyes. Dancers know, and have known for many millennia, that maintaining eye contact with a man holds him in a spell. It makes him feel as if, during that three- or four-minute private dance, she is his. Strippers and other exotic dancers allow men to live out the fantasy of choosing a young, beautiful woman to be his erotic consort or, in modern language, his fantasy girl—at least for a moment in time.

Dancers also provide a safe space in which a man can be his all-male, flesh-ogling self without fear of retribution or judgment. The dancer is there for him, and she is in the same establishment with him. They are partners in the taboo.

The Best Enjoy It

I once observed a dancer in a strip club in Honolulu, Hawaii, who had such an effect on men that I could barely believe she was just working. The men for whom she danced were almost sick with lust after she interacted with them. I noticed that no matter what movement she used to entice, she never lost eye contact.

She would get up close, her petite, dark-skinned body almost right on top of a guy and in his face, and look deep into his eyes. She'd move up and down and around him, constantly teasing him with her nipples, placing them ever-so-close to the man's mouth. She teased him mercilessly with her breasts. They weren't large, yet she presented them as if they were made for a man's pleasure (no touching allowed, however!). She seemed to shower her customers with her sexual energy. It was as if she were, metaphorically speaking, reaching into a man's soul and his pants simultaneously. I watched as one guy after another was drawn to her, waited his turn for the experience, and then was blown away by her performance. She was raking in the bucks for her efforts— and enjoying herself at the same time.

When I ran into her in the ladies' room later, I complimented her on her style and asked her how she felt about her work. I found her to be a very sincere young woman with a great attitude. She was a real person, a single mom with a kid at home and a boyfriend who lived on the north shore of Oahu.

"When I am working, I really am there with a guy," she told me. "I enjoy being in that moment. It's my job to serve his fantasy, but I am usually trying also to serve my fantasy. He probably has a wife and he'll go back to her horny and happier after being with me; and I have a boyfriend whom I love. But in that moment the man I am dancing for and I share a basic human connection. Because we are connected by our eyes, it is almost a soul connection. It doesn't work with every guy. I can't do it with men I think are hateful. But with the average, nice guy who comes into the club, I think: Okay, for a few minutes, I can love this guy and share a moment in time with him."

Not every professional exotic dancer is as gung ho about her work, nor does every stripper take a spiritual or artistic approach. Some strip environments are seedy, tacky, and disrespectful toward women; some dancers find their clients to be vulgar and vile. However, there are many strippers who enjoy their work, and there are many, many valid insights into seduction and titillation to be gained from women who dance for a living. In fact, extracting tips by watching exotic dancers is almost a sure thing. Think of it this way: Men have been paying for it for ages. It works! Why not look for elements to include in your own personal dance of seduction and your unique Seduction Signature! The most important thing to watch if you take a field trip to a strip club is how a man responds when a woman is dancing for him. If you could bottle it, you'd have him eternally under your spell.

The Seduction of Dance

While Gypsy Rose Lee, Jennie Lee, Dixie Evans, and other burlesque-style strippers are considered pioneers of the strip business, they'd be shocked and delighted to see the huge spectrum of entertainment that exists in that industry today— from your corner strip bar to elegant men's clubs to the female-friendly, sex-positive, woman-run Lusty Lady in San Francisco.

No matter what the medium, men have adored the sensual experience of having women dance for them for eons. From ancient times Indian women were taught the "Dance of Enticement," in which they swivel and swerve their hips, while using their hands, heads, and eyes to lure men. The Etruscans, who helped build the Roman culture, were known to revel in the sight of the naked female form in motion, having beautiful slave girls do gymnastics naked in front of them and with men. Middle Eastern cultures have for eons enjoyed the sensual rhythm of the belly dancer, who, no matter her size, proudly bares her naked midriff as she speaks to men with her writhing body and her enticing eyes. Many dances meant to arouse or entertain men rely as much on the eyes as on the flesh. For instance, belly dancers usually have a veil across their mouths, making the eyes the prominent facial feature.

Today, the allure of the exotic dancer is still a major turn-on for men. I hung out one evening at Tens—a classy, European-style exotic dancing club in Manhattan—to research what it is that gets men so gaga when naked women dance for them.

The place was packed with men in suits watching blondes in G-strings who danced on stages and pedestals and who, for twenty bucks, would do a private dance. (In less European-style places, they call them table dances.) Some of the chairs and tables had miniplatforms or stools the dancer could pull out and stand on to do a little breasts-in-your-face or at least close-to-your-tie, hip-swiveling, arm-swerving, sexually oriented entertainment.

At intervals, the women would step up to the stage to strut their stuff and the deejay would announce, essentially, that they were coming into the audience to privately tantalize anyone who dared to ask for a private dance; sometimes they offered two-for-one specials. Often, a woman would boldly go up to a guy with a smile and ask the polite equivalent of "Dance, Mister?"

In this elegant environment, filled with many truly beautiful women who had exceptionally well sculpted forms, I couldn't imagine a guy being able to say no to one of them. I never even realized that part of the fun was the fact that a guy could blow women off in this place and still have a gaggle more show up to ask the same question; it was a safe environment for a man to reject a beautiful woman and be assured she was not the last. In this environment, a man was King of the Castle, selecting a woman from his harem at whim. I marveled as these men observed the females and made their selections; it was much like a primal mating dance, but the search was not for a mate—it was for a fantasy.

A handsome, twenty-something guy sitting against the wall

waited and watched for the one he wanted; as a chorus line of ladies snaked across the floor, he tapped on the shoulder of the woman he'd quietly selected, summoning her over. She was petite and wild-looking, of some sultry Latin or European heritage with long dark hair, deep dark eyes, and exotic sensuality. She seemed so open and authentic, I could swear she was really digging on this cute young guy. When she danced for him, she maintained deep, sensual eye contact and, it seemed, made him feel that the only penis in the room for her was his. He gazed at her with a kind of unadulterated passion and admiration that made it seem as though they were intimates, lovers, connected beings.

I later asked him what made him choose her, how long he'd had his eye on her, and how he felt when he was looking at her that way. "It wasn't planned," he said, "but as she passed, I realized she was the look I wanted, that she was hot. I'm normally a very shy person, but I feel freer here, like I have permission to do this. You know when it's happening it's her job and she's going to be on to the next guy, so you never really feel like she's yours. But you can fantasize, for those few moments, that she is."

If men have been willing to pay for women to dance for them for eons, and keep coming back for more, it is clearly an art form of erotic expression that merits some study and participation. First of all, any man who loves to live out an occasional fantasy with a stripper will love any girlfriend or wife who gleefully lets him do that. A strip club is essentially a sacred space for men, yet your guy might enjoy a partner who accompanies him to see the dancers in action.

Temptress Traits to Emulate

Here are some traits of the exotic dancer that you can use without having to get a job as a stripper.

Eye contact. A professional dancer who knows how to utilize her body for the purpose of arousing men also knows how to hold a man under her spell with her eyes. Although men love the privilege and opportunity to blatantly stare at naked female flesh, it is the eyes that create the intimate man-to-woman connection. Connecting with the eyes is a way of reaching out and touching a man without having to say a word.

Visual tease. Since the art of the striptease is an experience of slowly removing clothing until there is very little left to the imagination, the first thing a good stripper learns is timing. She knows that if she just took her clothes off, a guy would think he's home with the wife, getting ready for bed—yawn! The slow, seductive, and artful removal of clothing one piece at a time holds a man's attention and builds up his desire.

Body comfort. Men prefer to be around women who like (or at least accept) their own bodies, and women who dance are usually quite secure in their own flesh. I've seen strippers who are chubby (not in New York, but in the Midwest), and dancehall girls who are really large and sporting really bad Frederick's of Hollywood knock-offs, and they all seemed totally at home, half or fully naked and otherwise exposed and vulnerable. Any woman who feels shame about her own body could benefit from exposure to women who do it for a living. Chances are the strippers had to get past their own inhibitions to reach the comfort zone or else they have a belief system that does not link their naked flesh with any negativity. Wouldn't you like to ask an exotic dancer (porn star, nude model) with a less-than-perfect body how she is able to do it?

Sexual self-expression. Watch a good stripper do her routine, and you will be wowed by her authentic sexual expression on stage. It pours out of her and onto the men. In exchange, money pours out of their pockets and gets tucked into the dancer's garter. Women who dance for men represent the kind of unabashed female sexuality that men hunger for—and that many women wish they had the courage to express. Dancers make it seem easy—but many will tell you that even for them it is a process of expanding their comfort level and trying new things. Others say they detach and simply "go away" when they are dancing (not recommended for budding seductresses who want to connect with their mates!).

Movement. A female body in motion is an enticing sight to the average man. That's why men go to dance clubs and strip joints to watch beautiful women dance, slither on stage, and hump poles. The moves that these women have are among the most erotic moves known to mankind, and they can be replicated in your own home. Swivel the hips, grind, strut, jut, press, push, hump, stretch...even those who think they can't can with a little practice. It's important to note: Any female body in motion in a sensual way will entice. Size and shape have little to do with sensuality; a three-hundred-pound women can look sexy as hell if she struts herself around with the proper attitude!

Allowing fantasies. Women who dance for a living offer a safe space for men because they allow them to have their fantasies. Men need to express that part of themselves in a place where they will not be judged or expected to perform. Couples can use strip clubs as foreplay. Let your guy go out and have a little fun; when he comes home, *you* reap the benefits.

Want to Be a Stripper Just for Fun?

Your assignment, should you choose to accept it:

- Go to a nice, safe neighborhood strip club—or visit one next time you're out of town—and see how the women dance and how the men respond.
- Observe what's called a table dance or private dance. This is when the dancer performs for an audience of one, rather than

onstage. The cost is generally $15 to $25, and the dance lasts for the length of one or two songs. Just watch how the man connects with the woman and maintains eye contact. It is an unbelievable sight!

💜 Rent *Striptease, Showgirls,* and *Blaze* to see how the pros learn to do it and how they perform when they are really into it. The physical performances in all are impressive! Rent *9½ Weeks* (with Kim Basinger and Mickey Rourke) to see how an amateur does it for her man and how he responds! Here is a list of Hollywood role models to learn from:

Rhonda Fleming in *Little Egypt* (1951)
Jayne Mansfield in *Too Hot to Handle* (1960)
Natalie Wood in *Gypsy* (1962)
Valerie Perrine in *Lenny* (1974)
Lolita Davidovich in *Blaze* (1989)
Elizabeth Berkley in *Showgirls* (1995)
Demi Moore in *Striptease* (1997)
Indira Varma in *Kama Sutra* (1997)

💜 Play some hot music and dance in the sexiest way you can. If you are inspired, toss off some garments as you go along. See how you feel. You might even find it a fun way to exercise!

8

Lessons From the Dominatrix

I'm a ba-a-a-a-d boy.
—Lou Costello, in all of his films

A dominatrix—also known as a domina, mistress, and fantasy engineer—is a sexually dominant woman who specializes in the erotic stimulation of men who enjoy being overpowered, controlled, and ordered around by women.

More often than not, a dominatrix is a true participant of the D&S scene and sees her work as an extension of her lifestyle choice. Sometimes she prefers to be known as a domina—for it signifies that she is sexually dominant in all of life, not just in her work. Almost always she is addressed as "Mistress." She demands gifts and service from her men (be they clients or lovers), and she is totally in charge of the show. The man is considered a slave, a submissive, a bottom.

Oftentimes these men are stimulated by being spanked, whipped, tied up, chained, and deliciously tortured with any manner of verbal and physical tactics. Sometimes they just like the idea of letting a woman take over.

A professional dominatrix usually charges upward of $150 an hour to sexually dominate a man. She sees him in her "dungeon," equipped with all sorts of domination tools. (Dungeon is typically the name of any playground where submissives and dominants can act out fantasies.) She doesn't have intercourse with him. She doesn't socialize with him. She makes his fantasy of total submission to a woman come true.

The game is that she is a woman revered, and he is a man not worthy of her personal passion. There is much proving of one's character in order for a bottom to earn the right to give sexual pleasure to the dominatrix, and even then it is totally on her terms. Part of the seduction is that she keeps him in a constant state of arousal and anticipation, and he never knows what will happen next!

In exchange, and in addition to paying her, he will shine her boots, massage her feet, or let her use his back as a chair. The core of the dominatrix-and-submissive behavior is that he worships, serves, and fetes her, and often buys her presents, and she willingly receives.

One of the true skills of a dominatrix is the same skill possessed by great strippers and women who have known how to work men throughout history—the ability to tease a man mercilessly and keep him in the game by giving him a little whiff but never quite letting him have the prize.

Don't feel guilty. As Mistress Tara Indiana, a New York domina, points out, many men are more in love with the idea of winning the prize than with actually winning it. They don't want the game to ever end. "Men want what a woman has between her legs," she says. "You have to make it like the part of you they will never have.

Tease them with it, but make them think you're never really going to give it up."

Powerful Women Never Pay

One of the hallmarks of the dominatrix-slave relationship is that it is *his* responsibility to prove his devotion to her by purchasing gifts, paying her bills, giving her money.

"Part of being a mistress, or having a mistress attitude, is knowing you can buy it for yourself, but letting him know that if he doesn't get it for you, somebody else will," Mistress Tara says. Letting men know you have expensive tastes is part of the game of letting them know you value yourself and they should too. It's a concept that is perfectly applicable to any relationship.

"If something is on sale, buy it yourself," she says. "Don't ever let him think he can buy you cheap things." It's the same principle as not grabbing the check on the first date because it will make him think you'll be doing all the paying.

There must be something to this philosophy because the D&S scene is flourishing, at least in New York. It has been featured in major stories, such as a 1995 exposé in *New York* magazine, and an S&M theme restaurant recently opened in Manhattan. Mistress Tara says she sees powerful guys plunk down fortunes to visit domination parlors and sex clubs. An entire universe in which the female rules exists out there. Her size, shape, age, and whether or not her breasts are still pert and pretty don't matter. She is revered. Even the female slaves are revered and cared for, because without a slave, a master has no game!

It's Fun Being a Dom Dame!

Acting like a dominatrix is fun. You can wear whatever you want, speak as you wish, and give men orders because that's what they have come to you for. My personal interpretation is you don't have to humiliate and cause pain to others to be sexually dominant—

well, maybe in small doses, for the purpose of teasing—but you do have to be a courageous, creative, and confident tease.

I like the dress-up aspect. It's fun to slip into slinky, revealing outfits that make you feel sexy and hot, because you in turn project sexual heat and confidence. For instance, a woman can have a fashion breakthrough just by wiggling into a leather bustier that pushes the breasts into her face and his and cinches the waist with Victorian precision, because it is just so decadent! While skyscraper-high pumps are not easy to navigate with on the streets of Real Life, I relish the idea of walking around with an attitude and air of confidence as my tantalized love-mate listens adoringly to the click of my heels.

Most of all, it turns me on to think that codependence might be cured when women come to understand that some men like to give up control and be dominated by a powerful female. And that it's time for women to stop feeling so guilty about treating men who ask for it like the true submissives they long to be.

As one of the few people who loved the film *Exit to Eden,* I was inspired by the concept of female sexual dominance as a lifestyle choice. Although I still don't see myself as a whip-wielding, chop-busting, humiliation queen, I like the idea of taking charge of sex. I like the idea of asking for what I want—and, well, taking it! It's been my experience that men like that too.

The more I look at it, the more I believe the dominant-submissive relationship is a metaphor for how the world works: There are tops and there are bottoms, and when you understand the core of who people are and how they operate, you can deal more effectively in the world. For instance, your boyfriend the CEO may be the boss all day and enjoy a little submissive play after work. You as the sexually dominant woman can bring him out and train him to be the woman pleaser you've dreamed of.

In my observation, people don't mess around as much with women who exhibit a sexually dominant nature. Sometimes it's out of a sense of respect or fear—the feeling that you never quite know what she'll do or say, so why rock her boat and risk getting your ego squashed. Some men find sexual confidence in women so alluring that it's almost frightening, and it throws their balance off. Or they get turned on in a productive way to women who can match wits and, it may seem to them, testosterone levels; many men love women who can be great sparring partners and still be feminine.

On Dominating Men

Other than a little erotic spanking game from time to time, games of bondage and discipline have never really banged the gong for me, but I love the idea of having the knowledge and skills to play them. It's like studying karate and feeling the power of your abilities, even if you never get to hip-throw Chuck Norris.

The social graces and interpersonal relationship skills of a mistress are also enchanting because she rules her environment and even keeps a globe on hand to indicate she's in control of her universe—mistress of her domain. For instance, sexually dominant women don't mince words, they don't walk around apologizing for being powerful, and they don't engage in the kind of codependent behavior that so many women today are so stuck in. They are less likely to be bullied by men because they don't see themselve as victims available for such abuse.

When a sexually dominant woman comes across surly men — you know the ones: rude, mean, militant, angry, seemingly unchangeable in their attitude, who try to make women feel powerless in their presence—she knows the proper way to view them is as boys in men's suits who are begging for some sort of discipline. This translates sexually, socially, and in business. Having had my share of relationships with guys who fed their own power by trying to strip me of mine, it's refreshing to realize that what they were really looking for was a good whack on the butt.

Now I know how to do it without feeling guilty and without even lifting a hand. As I said before, it's all in the attitude—because threatening, nagging, and begging never works with guys like that.

The attitude is, essentially, "Down on your knees when you speak to me." One way to achieve that is to take a deep breath, straighten your posture, maintain intense eye contact, and physically get into his space. Professional mistresses know how to communicate their displeasure to a man with just the click of their heels. Another powerful way to get a message across to an unruly male is with silence—it gets them every time.

A Field Trip to a Dungeon

The mistress, togged in a flesh-hugging black rubber dress, purposefully circled the male who knelt before her. All you could hear was the click of her five-inch heels on the slate floor of the "dungeon" and the sound of her breath. She lifted a lit cigarette to pouty red lips and tossed back her long, red mane as she sucked in a drag. As she inhaled, her elegant bone structure seemed even more pronounced in the dim light; her features formed a sexy, hard-edged look. There was something about the slight crook in her nose that made her look like a woman who could get nasty. She blew out the smoke and simultaneously flicked an ash, using the man's naked back as an ashtray.

"Where are you, baby?" she cooed in a loving voice.

"In your dungeon, Mistress," he responded quickly, nervously.

"And who owns this dungeon?"

"You do, Mistress."

"And who owns everything in this dungeon?"

"You do, Mistress."

"Then who owns you?"

"You do, Mistress."

She took another long drag, circled to his other side, hoisted up her dress slightly, and squatted, legs wide apart, right in front of his face. We could see the flesh of her sex and pubic hair through her white pantyhose—and he could too. She moved forward, brushing one of her large, luscious breasts against his head, and reached for his penis. Over his underwear, she touched it ever so lightly.

"And whose is this, baby?" she asked, brushing her hand over it.

"Yours, Mistress." He was practically panting now.

Abruptly, she rose, folded her arms across her chest the way angry mothers do, and positioned herself before him. Her black high-heeled shoes were level with his eyes as she scolded him.

"If it's mine," she said, suddenly stern and serious, "then why isn't it erect?"

Stunned silence permeated the room.

"Sorry, Mistress," he said, vowing to correct the situation. "I will do whatever you want me to do to get it that way."

This scene was part of a twelve-week training course on the art of being a sexually dominant woman, led by Mistress Tara Indiana, who promised to "whip" me into a dominatrix in no time. After going through her domination ritual, she turned to her students, all aspiring mistresses eager to try out some of these techniques at home, and explained that a submissive man should be erect just from looking at his mistress; that a man can be trained to get turned on just by the sound of a woman's clicking heels, or the scent of her perfume. Just the lilt of a woman's voice can make him rise to the occasion!

As for the guy on all fours—don't let his position fool you. Like many men attracted to sexually dominant women, he reveled in the opportunity to play with women who make the rules, call the shots, and administer sexual thrills from a position of supreme power. He was more than happy to be a guinea pig for the night.

He was totally seduced, elated, and satisfied by the experience.

If you think it's odd that a grown man would bow before a grown woman and present himself as a "slave," you would probably be even more amazed to know that some of the most powerful men on the planet find sexual domination one of the most delightful forms of seduction! The biggest suprise might be to find yourself enjoying the role of a woman who knows how to use a whip. Like karate, you may never need it in real life, but knowing you can do it gives you a sense of security!

More Than Just a Bonding Experience

Honing your skills as a sexual dominant is more than just learning about bondage and domination. Sure, you learn how to handle a whip, work a paddle, and give a meaningful spanking; how to tie a Boy Scout knot and lasso a pair of legs. You also need tutoring in techniques known to totally tantalize men—the key being the balance between teasing and surrendering, taunting and allowing, giving a man what he wants a little bit at a time and letting him beg for more.

During my studies, I ventured to the wildest adult clubs in New York—the Vault and Wildfire—and discovered a universe in which sexually dominant women rule. I also discovered, once you learn to accept your own power, others around you do too. And they want to do things for you.

During my training in domination, I went about my business in my usual manner and did not wear leather getups or carry whips to work (I was the editor in chief of *Playgirl* at the time). But I could see a significant shift in my attitude, just by the way men were responding to me—opening doors, asking to help me, picking up the tab pretty regularly, etc. The ultimate occurred during a downpour in New York City. I was waiting for a cab on a hugely busy street. A guy stood close by who I thought was going to fight me for a taxi. As it turned out, he hailed a cab *for me,* ran across the street to hold it for me, and then sent me on my way wishing me a good night!

In general, men seemed to no longer even bother to offer me meat-and-potatos sex dates, or even dinner and a movie, for that matter. But I entertained a lot of requests from men who wanted to kneel at my side, massage my feet, be my slave, or worship me in any way I might desire.

Learning From a Professional

Training with Mistress Tara was especially fun because she blows the image of the modern dominatrix—clad in leather and carrying the tools of the trade—out of the water. She encouraged students to discover their own particular attitude and M.O.—whether it be that of cheerleader with a whip or Bitch Goddess with a feather duster, or something in between.

"Not every mistress is mean," she says, explaining that she feels a dominant woman should always be a class act. Cool, smooth, professional, and conscientious, she never conducts herself like a man-hating bitch. "In fact, I like men," she says, "which is perhaps different than many dominatrixes, who often hate men."

She doesn't even call herself a dominatrix—"because that suggests someone who exclusively gets paid to do it"—she likes to be known as a *domina*. That's someone who lives the lifestyle and gets paid for it.

The thing that really drew me to Tara's course was that she appeared to be a walking advertisement for traits women can use anywhere, from the dungeon to the bedroom to the boardroom: lots of personal power, confidence in all her skills, and comfort in dominating her universe. She dressed sexy all the time—even her business attire was hot, worn with extremely high heels and pantyhose with no underwear. She made no bones about utilizing her sexuality to get what she wanted in life—and I don't mean screwing her way to the top. It's more about being the top.

During class, she showed us the proper way for a sexually dominant woman to sit—always with the chair back in front, between spread legs, with arms draped powerfully over its top. She was never, ever shy about the intimate display, à la Sharon Stone, that she often had on view for all to see.

To me, those things spelled power—power to both invent and control an environment by mastering it. Although sexual in nature, the power of the sexually dominant female transcends sexual situations and can be applied to all of life.

Temptress Traits to Emulate

Here are some temptress traits from sexually dominant women. I've culled some of the finer points, and they do not require the use of restraints or rope!

The power of the feminine. Being (or acting like) a dominatrix is just another way for a women to claim, express, and acknowledge her power and sexual prowess. In a culture that really only empowers women on the surface, it is a way for a female to take charge and communicate comfort with their sexual choices.

Control over sex. A dominatrix is not too shy to become skilled at sex play that turns her on. Being the predator or huntress of men can be fun. It's also fine to switch roles and play submissive, captive, and vulnerable parts. Sexual power is also choosing what you want to be, and when. Just make sure your partners are of the same mind. Even dominant men like women who take charge sexually. They're tired of always having to be the predators and performers. They enjoy a little seduction, or even a well-planned evening of sexual suprises.

Control over life. Just as you take the dominant role in a scene, those skills will help you take control of any situation. Sexual dominance can be a metaphor for empowering every aspect of your life.

Bargaining power. People do not argue with a woman with a whip in her hand. Metaphorically speaking, nobody messes with someone they perceive to be armed. Your confidence and your attitude are your greatest weapons. Generally, men are easily disarmed by a sexually confident woman—they may secretly resent you for it, but they'll give you what you want.

Being tops. People who are submissive choose to be that way. When you first train as a mistress, you begin to see that they are literally asking for it. Men hire women to dominate them and seek mates who will dominate them sexually because they like it. They are not really slaves, or victims. Some people are tops, some people are bottoms, and some people are what they call "switchables," but no one in the world of the dominatrix is there unless they want to be. The great part is that everyone is free to play as they choose.

Fun and games. Women who learn to think on their feet can come up with some tantalizing sexual tricks. Merciless teasing with all your body parts, the use of delightfully sexy clothes and props, and fun with sex toys can win big points in the boudoir.

Sexuality as a metaphor for real life. Just as you get a rush when you ski down your first slope, taking a sexual risk can be invigorating and can open up many areas of your life. As I said, you never have to even lift that whip, but knowing you can do it, and realizing that there are many men who would love you to do it, gives you a certain confidence that can be translated into all areas of life.

Want to Be a Dominatrix Just for Fun?

Your assignment, should you choose to accept it:

- Choose a dominant dame as a role model. Here are some suggestions from the film world:

Myrna Loy in *The Mask of Fu Man Chu* (1932)

Raquel Welch in *The Magic Christian* (1969)
Laura Antonelli in *Venus In Furs* (1982)
Kathleen Turner in *Crimes of Passion* (1984)
Dana Delany in *Exit To Eden* (1994)

- ♥ Consider taking an adult education course on this topic or putting a group of friends together and visiting an S&M club. There are a number in New York—the Vault, Hellfire, the Eulenspeigel Society—that are safe and friendly. For out-of-town locations, try calling one of those New York clubs for a lead.

- ♥ Observe what goes on in the scene. The players in this community are generally normal people who like to come out and play. There is an extraordinary amount of respect and privacy; the sex clubs, in fact, are tenacious about protecting their patrons from invasions of privacy as well as protecting themselves from anyone in the club who does not follow the rules. Hellfire has "S&M police," bouncers who break up any indiscretions in a heartbeat.

- ♥ Go to a sex shop and try out a whip. You might find great freedom and delight in whisking it through the air and hitting a wall or the floor. You can always buy it and take it home to practice.

- ♥ Practice saying the Mistress Mantra in the mirror until you feel it's part of you: "Down on your knees before you speak to me!"

9

Lessons From the Sexpot

> If a woman hasn't got a streak of harlot in her
> she's as dry as a stick as a rule.
> —D. H. Lawrence

Beyond the femme fatale, dominant dame, and dancer, there is a breed of seductive beauty known as the sexpot.

Anyone can be a sexpot because this is the most generic and easy-to-emulate form of female sexual self-expression. The sexpot is a woman who is so in touch with her own sexuality that men can't miss it. She so clearly owns her feminine nature that it pours out of her. Sensuality surrounds her like an aura and a scent. She is all about seduction and allure.

Her time-honored traditions—the swivel of the hips as she walks, the suggestive show of cleavage, the wink of the eye, the come-hither stare, the sometimes bold sexual gestures—have been passed on through generations. We've seen her in Mae West, Marilyn Monroe, Jayne Mansfield, and Madonna.

Yet the sexpot is not just the in-your-face lady of lust. She is also the shy and demure dame who bats her eyelashes and drops her hanky, the woman who gently, or perhaps innocently, puts forth the suggestion of seduction and smoothly lures a man to her (Andie MacDowell, for instance). She is the damsel in distress who lets a guy be the big, tough caveman who saves her, yet she is a smart damsel who doesn't give away her power in the process. Lois Lane, for example, snags Superman by: 1. believing in him and being someone he can trust, and 2. playing a seemingly demure damsel to his save-the-world champion. Yet she's still able to kick ass at her day job as a tough reporter, and both behaviors are authentic.

The sexpot is also a woman who is so sexy that she's slightly dangerous. Think of all the babes in James Bond movies, such as Pussy Galore, the leather-clad character played by Honor Blackman in *Goldfinger.* They are always women who exude sex, and danger, and 007 likes them that way!

The sexpot comes in so many varieties that we don't even have names for all her many faces and facets, but here are just a few variations: She's the sexy siren, the blond bombshell, the saucy vixen, the vamp, slutty girl, fast woman, sex kitten, damsel in distress, and Lolita. The common thread among sexpots is they are genuine in their brand of sensual self-expression, and they are, quite obviously, irresistible to men.

Sexy Sirens

The sirens, mythical singing creatures of ancient Greece who were half woman and half bird, would seduce sailors on the seas with their irresistible voices. These daughters of Neptune would force seamen off course and cause them to crash into their island. In the *Odyssey,* Odysseus plugged his ears with wax and tied himself to the mast of his ship to avoid succumbing to the sweet temptation of the sirens' song.

The use of the term siren originates from those mythical creatures, but today it is used to describe women who are considered irresistible: supermodel Elle McPherson, actress Pamela Anderson Lee, singers Mariah Carey and Toni Braxton. The original sirens were seen as dangerous, and our culture still perceives an irresistible woman as a bit of a threat to a man. Let's face it, sirens scare everyone a little, because when men find a woman irresistible, they lose control in the onslaught of hormones. (Think of what Michael Douglas's fatal attraction to Glenn Close did to him!)

Obviously, the modern seductress doesn't want to be that dangerous to her man. But the Sirens demonstrated something that most women long to emulate: the ability to seduce men through a no-fail method of enticement; i.e., they knew the seductive magic of their own voices. I believe any woman can be a Siren by picking one thing about herself that she knows is a sure thing and focusing on it.

As actress Yasmine Bleeth told me: "Everyone has something that's beautiful—whether it's her breasts or butt, or beautiful arms, legs, shoulders, or back. Show off your best assets."

Whether it's a body part or a special talent, the way you move, or the way you dress, focus on what you do have and utilize it. Work it, girl! You may not sing, but perhaps you have a way of whispering in a guy's ear that drives him wild, of giving him a special come-hither look, or dressing in a way that he can't ignore.

The sirens, singing was a natural form of self-expression. It poured from them with beauty and grace. As you explore the many approaches of classic seductresses, think: What's natural for me? If you enjoy a certain form of self-expression, you are more likely to find your man responding with all-male delight. When that happens, it is evidence that you are being all the siren you can be.

The Blond Bombshell

Think Mae West. While she is in a category unto herself, she is also part of a long line of sexy women who relied on peroxide and moxie to make their point to the world: "I'm sexy. I'm expressing it. Get out of my way if you don't like it." Marilyn Monroe, Jayne Mansfield, and the most recent icon to resurrect the blond bombshell, Madonna, all share that in-your-face quality of seduction.

When a woman like this enters a room, her sensuality comes with her...no, it comes in before her and it fills a room like smoke. Because her sexuality is projected so far out there, it touches people. It stirs them up. It creates a sense of longing and desire. That's why men often appear to be so hopelessly eager around blond bombshell sexpots. They feel as if all their senses— and sense of control—have been taken over. But don't worry...they like it. As Mae West once said, "Women with pasts interest men because they hope history will repeat itself!"

Fast Women and Slutty Girls

"I want a date with one of those Jersey girls. They wear black pointy bras and white lipstick. They do naughty things...like let you smell them all over." That's how Jonathan Silverman, in *Stealing Home,* sums up why boys like slutty girls.

Slutty women are irresistible to men because they represent the ultimate taboo. They are the girls you can't take home to Mom but whom you want all the other guys to know about. Slutty girls and their counterpart, fast women, make no bones about boners. They are all about wanting sex, and men want to be around babes who ooze lust.

A slutty girl's motto is "Why wait and why worry?" She can range from an ultrafeminine lady dressed in a skimpy, sexy outfit—your basic short skirt, low-cut shirt, high heels—to a tough, almost mannish dame who enjoys men without apologies.

Take the character Rizzo in *Grease,* for example. Stockard Channing portrayed her has a tough-as-nails high school babe who hid her vulnerability underneath her sexual conduct—and occasional misconduct. Yet she sang a song about how her sexuality was so misunderstood: "There are worse things I could do, than go with a boy or two." She had a rep for being fast, but the guys loved that. In a way, she was one of them.

Slutty girls and fast women are a staple of American movie culture, and are often portrayed as less-than-admirable bimbos. Nevertheless, there is an entire subculture of women who love that slutty look—just go to the mall and take a peek inside a Frederick's of Hollywood store. In certain parts of the country, big hair, big cleavage, tight jeans, short skirts, and blatant showing of skin are the norm.

With slutty girls, men feel sexually confident in their ability to turn a woman on—because she is already turned on when they get to her—and they are able to relax because they know they are going to get sex without having to work so hard!

Vixens and Vamps

Vixens and vamps exude a sexuality that lies somewhere between bombshell and slut, with a dash of dominatrix. The suggestion of sex is always there. They have a rather hard-hitting, come-hither quality that is a combination of openness and allure. Catwoman is a good example. She's pure sexuality with claws. She's seductive and sexy, and uses that to dominate and control. For the man who likes to be toyed with like a little catnip ball, a vixen/vamp like this is the cat's meow.

The vixen is like a wild cat, for her sensuality seems to growl at you. It is more untamed. The vamp can be otherworldly, like Vampira, or just a darker version of a vixen. Both sexpots speak to the male desire for a walk on the wild side and a peek at the dark side. For women who are not quite drawn to the dominatrix, yet like a slightly hard-edge approach to seduction, the vixen or vamp can be a fun sexpot to emulate.

Sex Kittens or Lolitas

Sex kittens almost automatically have that damsel-in-distress quality about them. Unlike the sexpots who love to navigate through the jungle of love, the sex kitten is more demure and receptive. She doesn't search out her man, she lures him right to her with what seems to be a naturally receptive female openness.

Barbarella is the ultimate sex kitten. While she has all the qualities of a siren and vixen, she doesn't flaunt or make a point about her sexuality. She simply lives in it, and men find her so appealing they have the need to pleasure her. And she gets into so much trouble as she travels through galaxies that men have the desire to rescue her. Ultimately, she is strong and she is in full charge of her sexuality—and she adores pleasure!—but the way she expresses it is pure sex kitten.

Ann-Margret, who made a movie called *Kitten With a Whip*, is also one of the classic sex kittens. In her movies, she's a seethingly sexy creature who is so sweet you can't consider her anything but a kitten. Demure, playful, sexy…she has the ability to draw men in with her smooth sex-kitten ways. See *Viva Las Vegas* to learn why Elvis was magnetized by her.

Lolita, the young girl who was Humbert Humbert's obsession in the literary work of the same name, is another type of sex kitten—a young girl whose coyly seductive charms reel a man in like a fish on a hook. Lolita speaks to a man's need for youth and freshness, his desire to be immortal, and his need to care for a woman. When men age and begin to feel their virility lagging, they seek a Lolita to pump up their testosterone level. The purr of any sex kitten can do that.

Temptress Traits to Emulate

The Siren

Music is a great way to inspire your own personal Siren. Find music that speaks to the voice within and let it bring you out. Mythology is another. Read about the mythical sirens, about the seductive Calypso (also in the *Odyssey*) and the goddesses of ancient Greece and Rome. The stories often depict enticing women and creatures who know their strength and power, who anticipate the results of their seduction, and hence get what they want. Some of these archetypes can be applied to daily life in simple ways. Knowing your strong seduction points and focusing on those points can bring you success!

The Blond Bombshell

Watch old blond bombshell movies, especially those of Mae West. Get a form-fitting glamour dress and practice the attitude walk. Try on a blond wig or, if you're daring and ready for a change, dye your hair blond. See how it feels to live like a blond bombshell.

Blond Bombshells in Film

Marilyn Monroe, *The Seven-Year Itch* (1955)
Brigitte Bardot, ... *And God Created Woman* (1956)
Jayne Mansfield, *Will Success Spoil Rock Hunter?* (1957)
Mae West, *Sextette* (1978)
Jessica Rabbit, *Who Framed Roger Rabbit?* (1988)

The Slutty Girl

Any woman who hungers to express that side of herself might find it useful to coax her out with sexy clothes. Get your hands on the sluttiest outfit you can find, the one that exposes more than you've ever exposed before, and meet your man out on a date, or at the door, looking like a fast woman. Meet him at a bar, dressed like a hooker or an extremely hot babe, and see what happens. Watch Melanie Griffith in *Something Wild* (1986) to get ideas.

The Vixen or Vamp

Rita Hayworth in *Gilda* is a favorite example of a world-class vixen in action. She is all about expressing her sexuality and seducing men. See the movie and try to find a retro dress like Hayworth's. Sometimes fabulous clothes will help change your attitude. Make sure you show lots of cleavage. Try playing the vixen at a costume party or an event where you can easily practice until you find out whether or not you have a true vixen spirit.

The Sex Kitten or Lolita

Baby dolls and teddies get the point across. So do short-shorts and shirts that tie under the breasts and show off the belly. Often the spirit of the sex kitten or Lolita comes through in a pout. And when a man sees that pout, he wants to make things better; when he sees those pursed lips, he wants to kiss them. Watch some sex-kitten or Lolita movies to get a sense of how men go wild around women who act slightly young, slightly spoiled, and slightly pouty.

Lolitas in Film

Sue Lyon, *Lolita* (1962)
Carrie Fisher, *Shampoo* (1975)
Jodie Foster, *Taxi Driver* (1976)
Rachel Ward, *The Thorn Birds* (1980)
Michelle Johnson, *Blame It on Rio* (1984)
Brooke Shields, *Pretty Baby* (1978)

PART III ❤

Making It Real

10

Overcoming Seduction Shyness

I'm a bit of a prude myself.

—Gypsy Rose Lee, famous burlesque-style
exotic dancer

As you sort through the images of seductresses past and present and consider how you might work elements of those pioneers of passion into your personal Seduction Signature, remember that it's supposed to be fun! Anything new is a challenge, but, trust me, you can be as hot and spicy as your favorite sexpot, do a private striptease for your man, and make it through without cracking up—or falling apart from nerves!

Even Gypsy Rose Lee had to start somewhere! And anyone who watches a Madonna music-video marathon can tell that her status as a supreme seductress was not very evident in "Like a

Virgin." Becoming the seductress you want to be takes time—and you are in the process of creating her every day.

While most of us come into the world with a childhood innocence and uninhibited nature that gives us freedom to dress up and be wild exhibitionists, studies show that most women lose it around age nine, when the realities of being female and the expectations for our gender set in.

We develop a painful awareness of our bodies and faces, our body parts and skin; and the unending assessment of what we are, and who we are not, begins. If you are reading this book, you may be one of those once-playful women who's been trying to find her way back to the free-spirited little girl who dressed in mom's shoes, loved playing with her makeup, and dug wearing boas, pearls, and fancy hats.

Part of overcoming seduction shyness and becoming bold is recapturing the spirit of a time when you were a natural seductress, because you simply exuded what you were, without judgment—you simply were who you were. The great part of recapturing the spirit of girlhood is that now you are a grown woman with permission to do whatever you want to do.

How Bold?

There's a saying that goes, "We teach what we most need to learn." That perhaps could apply to writer, sex educator, and cultural sexologist Carol Queen, an unabashed exhibitionist who devotes herself to teaching women how to assess their erotic I.Q.s and follow their fantasies toward more fulfilling sensual self-expression. It's almost impossible to believe that a woman as seemingly uninhibited as Queen was once painfully shy.

This was part of her impetus for documenting her charming techniques for other shy women in her 1996 book, *Exhibitionism for the Shy,* and for teaching workshops on dressing up, showing off, and talking hot, since 1991. Her students are composed of women seeking their inner seductresses and trying to develop a personal style.

"It's not about flashing," she explained to me. "It's about finding a place within you, and within what your limitations are; and, as you become more comfortable, to really have a good erotic time."

This is the key to the evolving seductress's journey: expanding your comfort level as you go along, adding new things as appropriate, and having a good time with whatever it is you are doing. Queen is the first to acknowledge that the art of exhibition takes a finely tuned and individual approach. The truth is, some seductresses want to become professional strippers—others just want to feel confident enough to stand naked in the shower with a lover!

Outing Your Seductress

"On one level, women are more encouraged to be more exhibitionist, taking special care in how we look, for example," Queen points out. "Yet, I think we also often labor under difficult erotic self-esteem issues. Together, those two things can create difficulty for women around exhibitionistic behavior."

To Queen, exhibition is about showing yourself off erotically in a way that makes you *feel* erotic. "Not everybody is turned on by the notion of being erotically outgoing, dressing sexier, masturbating in front of someone, or any of the various things that could fall under exhibitionism. But plenty of people who might be directed that way are really stopped by this erotic self-esteem issue. For people who would be inclined to explore eroticism more deeply, and yet their self-esteem is hanging them up, it would be a worthwhile issue to look at."

In the early nineties, Queen appeared in the famous video *How to Female Ejaculate,* sans clothing. In the video she masturbates and ejaculates for the camera, describing her experience as she goes along, with the comfort and ease of a casual dinner conversation. She seems totally at home naked or in sexy outfits, masturbating or showing her sexual self, and talking about it simultaneously. Her journey from shy girl to bold exhibitionist may be inspiring to the aspiring exhibitionist.

"I had been attracted to theater, dress-up, and establishing sort of a different persona, so I evolved this crazy wardrobe. I remember dressing up for my birthday in fishnets and a tailcoat when I was eighteen or nineteen, at a party where I was actually too shy to talk to all the people there. Yet I was projecting myself as being out there and very bold.

"Then, through eroticism with a partner with whom I felt safe, I began to conquer the shyness that overwhelmed me in other places. I finally found that part of myself. My partner liked that I was into this dress-uppy, bold thing and was willing to sort of walk with me through that process and encourage me. Gradually, I brought the bold, theatrical image into my real sex life. That's what really made a difference for me."

The process of becoming more of who you really want to be is ongoing. Each time you succeed, you gain power for the next time. "You go out there, or you're in your bedroom, and you do something that's more daring than you've ever done; you don't die, and you say, 'Oh, it works.'"

Queen says the best tip for shy people who are anxious to dress up but don't have the nerve is to wait until Halloween or Mardi Gras and find an appropriate place to try something different.

A Personal Tale

I waited a long time for my first opportunity to go out in public wearing a bustier (a black, corsetlike piece of lingerie that pulled in my waist and gave my breasts that in-your-face look). When I finally did, I thought, I'll never get away with this; I was sure the fashion police would bust me. I wore it to a rock-and-roll performance by the rocker guy who had broken my heart. My whole intention in dressing up was to be able to walk away as a proud seductress rather than as a shattered woman.

Mistress Tara (the professional domina I'd trained with), a woman totally in touch with her ability to dress up and devastate men, came to get me ready for the big night. She found me decked out in a denim jacket, cowboy boots, and ordinary clothing. She wouldn't let me leave the house that way. Thus, it was exhibitionist baptism by fire.

"You have to look devastating," she said. "You have to put tits in his face *and* be elegant. That is the only way to leave a guy like that."

She put my long hair in an elegant sweep and helped me wiggle into a black bustier that made my breasts look like they were an offering (in this case, one that would never be made to the mock star again). She talked me into wearing a long see-through skirt, beautiful maroon velvet jacket that seemed terribly flashy to me, and heeled boots. Even though I could not bear to wear the really spiky heels Mitress Tara urged me to try, I must say I was dressed to kill, and by wearing such a hot costume I *felt* like a man killer. The nice girl who let a guy step all over her was replaced by a hot woman who had the confidence to tell him to hit the road.

While I felt okay in my apartment, leaving the house for a noisy club was another thing. At the club, Tara and I met up with my good friend Dr. Judy Kuriansky and others, who came especially to support me during my big moment! As I watched the mock star's performance, I felt my own performance anxiety, knowing my friends and I would be going backstage after the show. I had so many eyes on me that I became self-conscious. I started smoking cigarettes out of nervousness and sipping a little more vodka than I'd intended to (not something I'd ever repeat, for that reason, or any other). When the moment of truth finally came, I stepped into a backstage dressing room, and Mr. Rocker's eyes bugged out of his head—truly, they did. He couldn't take them off me. Even though it was a night of utilizing my powers of seduction on a man I wanted *out* of my life (also not something I'd repeat), it was worth it to me to go out with a bang and get to wear a devastating outfit.

I've since learned my lesson about not keeping men I don't want under my spell. I utilize my most devastating looks for men I want to be with. But back then, it worked wonders. It was closure for me—to have his full attention and yet walk away with my pride and confidence in place.

Today I remember it as a moment in time in which my desire to empower my confidence overrode my fears of being rejected, laughed at, or, worse, going unnoticed. Having had my "exhibitionist moment" under tense conditions, I can say from experience that it will be smoother if you start out with an exhibitionist moment that is not emotionally loaded, and gear your best seductive stuff toward someone you do want to seduce. That way, dressing to devastate can be great fun!

The Novice Exhibitionist

Public exhibition is a challenge at first—under any conditions. Often, you develop an extraordinary awareness of your own flesh and posture and any little discomfort gets exaggerated and becomes a focal point. Queen agrees, it's not uncommon to feel goofy and weird when you're in the beginner stage. There is, however, a way to practice.

Queen suggests the following:

- Start with things that are sexier than what you wear now, but, in your opinion, not outrageous. Any of us can think of a range of erotic outfits and decide, for example, to go with the lace teddy. Perhaps hold off on the bustier that makes your breasts look like they're on a shelf and the tight, black vinyl pants.

- Begin in the realm of your comfort level. There isn't any reason to take yourself all the way out to the end of the gangplank just because you're pushing yourself to get brave as fast as possible, unless that kind of push works for you as a matter of course—which is usually not the case with really shy people.

- Ease into the level of boldness that would take you in the *direction* of the black, skin-tight vinyl and the dominatrix garb. But start with items from Victoria's Secret, or whatever; and move at your own pace. If you have a partner who is encouraging you to become more outgoing, take him shopping.

The Discomfort Factor

I marvel at women who can keep their feet in five-inch heels and reveal their form in tight clothes. Even on a good day, with good intentions, I am not typically a high-heeled, tight-clothing kind of gal. I can barely walk in come-get-me pumps. In fact, I've long since traded the hard-edged bustier for a softer, more feminine Wonderbra look that still makes breasts look tempting but allows simple pleasures like breathing.

Not every woman is meant to wear skimpy clothes and high, high heels. It's important to know that every female can create her own seduction style, in terms of both a look or behavior.

Throughout history, women have sacrificed comfort for fashion and have literally deformed their bodies trying to be sexy, slimmer, and hot looking. Many women suffered spine problems and disfigurement from tight-fitting corsets that were such a common part of women's wardrobes in the 1700s and 1800s. But dressing up today is not supposed to do us in.

Queen recommends former X-rated film star Annie Sprinkle's workshop "Sluts and Goddesses" (also available on video) as a fabulous resource on this topic. There two different female sexual archetypes are explored, and each is considered and embraced as a viable option. There's the slut, in tight clothes, push-up bras, with rocket-cone-shaped breasts, and platform high heels. And then there's the goddess, in the sexy, lacy, flowing, comfortable, bejeweled, gorgeous fabric; a sort of spiritual sexual side. You'll notice the goddess archetype is very comfortably dressed, yet elegant and alluring.

Dressing sexy and being an exhibitionist is not always about revealing more flesh. As Queen explains it, "Sexuality clearly shines out from both the slut and the goddess. This means the woman who isn't interested in the tight push-up-bra kind of garments might find increased self-esteem if she tries the slinky, sheer-scarf look. People need to keep an open mind about what's sexy; don't be limited to the images of a Frederick's of Hollywood [catalog] or a fetish magazine. If something else works for you it will enhance your sexuality just because you feel sexier wearing it."

Queen believes women can have fun with their fantasies in a very healthy way. "Persona play doesn't necessarily mean splitting off into a whole separate personality, or encouraging yourself into multiple personalities," she points out.

For people who are really at the beginning of this process and are feeling kind of shy, they may find it useful to let that part of them take over for a little while. For example, if you think Linda Marie is insufficiently sexy and adventurous, call that part of yourself Trixie and let Trixie take over.

There is a force of energy in each and every one of us that isn't squashed by the way we've felt squashed by society and by other people's expectations; by our own performance anxiety and negative self image; a part that is braver than the rest. You can have fun wherever you are!

11

How to Be a Private Dancer

That's it, baby! When you got it, flaunt it. Flaunt it!
—Zero Mostel, _The Producers_

I have been a proponent of women stripping at home for their men since I took a stripping course that taught me to use the elements and the art of the striptease to bolster my courage in the boudoir.

I like to watch women dance and love to watch the way that men watch them. For fifteen years, I made a hobby of stopping by strip clubs around the country, in cities I happened to be visiting and in Mexico, to pick up the local flavor and study what it was that so aroused men when they were in those environments.

From Nashville to Acapulco, there is one common denominator—beyond naked flesh—that I found in every club: The captivated, mesmerized way a man looks at a woman who is dancing for him when she maintains eye contact. If only you could bottle that look—the passion, the lust, the adoration in a man's eyes—and take it home. Women might be suprised to see how intimate it can be, with men sometimes looking into the eyes of these strangers as if they were old lovers. It is magical. And the more I observed it during private dances, the more I came to understand that ultimately it doesn't matter if the body is perfect or if the dance is extraordinarily erotic. When the eye contact is there, the connection is made, and the fantasy flourishes!

Dancers who are fully engaged in and enjoying their own sensual self demonstrate enviable freedom and comfort in their own flesh, and they have a lot to teach about getting comfortable with exhibition; even the dancers who are detached, yet good at their craft, can demonstrate a few tricks. But I am convinced that the woman who masters eye contact and stays with it will triumph as an at-home stripper.

This takes pressure off of performance and puts emphasis on connecting. Just as the shedding of clothes will promise passionate things to come, your eyes can speak volumes about what's in store. If stripping for a party of one grabs you, consider domesticating this favorite sex sport at home: who knows...maybe he'll skip that night out with the boys for a private performance.

I'm not saying you shouldn't hone your seductive strip skills or have fun getting into sensual, expressive dancing, I am just pointing out that the pressure to time every step and be perfect does not exist at home. And yet, so many men would welcome the effort!

You may not be rushing out to buy those long, sexy gloves (to throw in his face as your strip) right now, but keep at-home stripping in mind. It grabbed me one night out of the blue when I was sitting in a strip club with two exotic dancers with impossibly cute names (Ecstasy and Brandy). I had shared a limo back from a

TV show with them, and they invited me and a friend in to see the club. We all sat together watching the multiple-stage activities, and one of the dancers, Ecstasy, an enthusiastic twenty-seven-year-old mom with a four-year-old daughter, took so much delight in seeing her buddies perform that she turned to me and said: "Oh, they're so good—doesn't it make you want to get up there and take off your clothes?"

It did—but I was far too shy to admit it at the time. It could be said that my interest in the strip world was fueled by my secret fantasy of being a private dancer for an audience of one—and feeling totally confident and sexy about it. I eventually made my fantasy come true—after a lot of practice. Had I known then what I know now about eye contact, I would have spent the time practicing staring into people's eyes rather than just practicing taking off my clothes.

"Look at Me, I'm Stripping!"

In 1988 I took a course called "How to Strip for Your Man" and it changed my life. I developed so much confidence in the company of the thirty other women of all shapes, sizes, and ages who were attempting to learn how to strip in a three-hour course that I went out and began being bolder and more assertive with men.

Held in the Radio City Hall dance studio, a fabulous teacher—then a B-film actress, now a Ph.D.—taught us every bump, grind, gyration, twist, turn, and move known to tantalize men. We practiced on a chair, and pretended it was our audience of one. We stripped clothes off, we put clothes on sexy, we learned the attitude walk.

After I finished the course, I was so turned on by the thought of stripping for my new boyfriend, that I decided to create a little routine for him. The problem was, I locked myself into a few props and ideas that were great for my stripping teacher but difficult for me. She was tall, leggy, and of perfect breasts and

I…well, I wasn't. She also wore stiletto heels as comfortably as slippers. I didn't.

The first time I ever practiced stripping, in a mirror, I put on sky-high shoes I couldn't walk in and wore a hat that wasn't me. I carried a cane that I'd used for my foot injury months before, and while it was fun to play with, it didn't feel quite right. Overall, I felt stupid and fat, and I couldn't imagine doing this routine for my audience of one. I was disappointed because I really wanted to strip for my guy. I knew that I enjoyed many of the moves and I felt that I had the sex appeal to carry it off. All I needed was a confidence boost—and a few adjustments.

A few practice sessions later, I realized the shoes just didn't work for me, and the hat…well, it would take some getting used to. The cane, if replaced by an umbrella, was more palatable. Most important was that I realized I really loved to dance. The sensuality bubbled from inside me to the surface when I surrendered to the dancing. It was so much more fun to focus on the music (not the props or dance steps) and allow it to carry me into the mood. I spent weeks preparing my personal "stripping tape"—songs I loved to move to. The tips I learned in stripping class were much easier to incorporate into my own natural body movements. I ditched the spikes for a more sensible, albeit less sexy, pair of shoes.

The night I finally stripped for my honey—months after my initial practice sessions—I felt as if the seductress in me was born. Like a spirit guide or guardian angel, she got me through the experience, performance anxiety and all! She helped me take baby steps to success! I wasn't a professional stripper, and I didn't try to be one. I was myself. I was nervous and shaky when I started, and I felt all the feelings of a stripper on her first time out. Yet being my sensual self—while dancing, stripping off clothes, and doing all sorts of tantalizing things—was quite a turn-on for the man in my life. He was beyond seduction. He was mine!

I incorporated something I wanted to learn how to do (stripping) with a fantasy of a way I wanted to be with a man (comfortable in my own skin and sexy in my movements), and did it in my own style.

While anyone certainly can, and should, learn some sexy dance steps from Demi Moore (star of *Striptease*), no one can *be* her. None of us should try. All of us, however, can have a shot at adapting any form of seductive expression to our own personal style. If you watch *Striptease* you might relate to a scene in which she is blow-drying her hair and just practicing some dance steps in the mirror—nice and natural, just for her.

You Can Do It, Too

If you have any desire to put on sensual music and sway to the beat, or if you are itching to strip for an audience of one, check out the movies listed in chapter 7, "Lessons From the Stripper," and consider going to a strip club; but feel free to just roll with whatever is inside you. Exotic dancer G. G. Long, who taught a successful strip course at the Discovery Center in New York, shared some special warm-up and strip tips with me.

Before you even begin to try a strip routine—as a practice run or for your guy—turn out all the lights and touch yourself from head toe. Sensually stroke your face, your nose, your lips, your breasts; touch your hips, your legs, your knees, your ankles, your toes. Go up and down, passing over your belly and your breasts. "Explore your own body," she says. "Touch it, feel it, arouse yourself. This will raise your energy and enthusiasm.

"Also, use erotica to get excited. Before you get with your man, you want to get with yourself. Watch a tape, listen to a video, read a hot book. Get your juices flowing so you are already in a state of excitement when you get out on your own personal dance floor."

While you are dancing for your man, try some of these tantalizing moves:

- ♥ Maintain eye contact as much as possible
- ♥ Communicate with your eyes and lips
- ♥ Arch your back, throw your hair back, caress your neck
- ♥ Use your nails to erotically scratch your legs, your butt, your tummy
- ♥ Lick yourself—anywhere your please
- ♥ Suck your finger, run it along your lip
- ♥ Lick your lips, keep your lips parted
- ♥ Caress yourself, anywhere
- ♥ Smack your own naked behind
- ♥ Glide your bare toes over his lips
- ♥ Move your legs against his chest
- ♥ Brush ever-so-slightly against his crotch
- ♥ Pinch his nipples with your toes
- ♥ Command his legs by wrapping yours around them
- ♥ Brush your breasts against his chest, over his shirt
- ♥ Brush your breasts against his chest when you take his shirt off
- ♥ When the time comes, open a condom packet by tearing it open with your mouth and look him boldly in the eyes

Bringing It Home

To prepare for your home-stripping debut, make sure all your props are at hand and your music is cued. It's best to use a prerecorded stripping tape that has all the songs in your routine. Have everything ready to go in the room or area you intend to use as a performance space.

Create the right mood with low lights or candlelight. Spray your favorite perfume into the air and play some soft, romantic music to set the tone. (For additional tips, see Chapter 13, "Creating the Environment.")

Your opportunity to strip could be the nightcap to a fun evening out, or it could be the start of a hot night in! Whichever the case, make sure that your man is relaxed and comfortable

The Music of the Night

G. G. Long says the following tunes are sure to complement the music you make with your man. Here's a play list that's popular among professional dancers. Try them out and incorporate your own favorites. Select whatever sounds set your dancing soul in motion!

For a Slow, Sensual Striptease:

- "Fire 'n' Desire," Rick James
- "Sexual Healing," Marvin Gaye
- "Little Red Rooster," Rolling Stones
- "Do Me Baby," Prince
- "Wonderful Tonight," Michael Bolton
- "Georgia," Michael Bolton
- "Secret Garden," Madonna
- "You Can Leave Your Hat On," Joe Cocker

For a Fast, Sizzling Strip:

- "Baby, You're a Star," Prince
- "Fever," Madonna
- "Love Toy," Gloria Estefan
- "Sexy Noises," Salt 'n Pepa
- "I'm So Excited," Pointer Sisters

before you proceed. This could mean cuddling and kissing, or even dancing together to start. It may be nothing more than taking off his jacket, loosening his tie, and enjoying a sip of wine together.

You can work your way into an impromptu striptease or begin more dramatically by announcing you are about to treat him to a very special performance—it depends on your personal style. Just make sure he's got a comfy seat and is not distracted (i.e., make sure there are no TVs or cellular phones to get in the way and you are not expecting any guests).

When a man watches a woman dance, he is often unabashedly turned on. He pays attention and focuses on the lust of the moment. He sits back and receives it as one who deserves to be danced for. Men have paid—for ages and ages—to see women remove their clothes, shake their breasts, touch themselves, gyrate their hips, tease, and tantalize them. So why not do it yourself, in the comfort of your own home? I wholeheartedly recommend you start dancing around the house and see how sexy you will feel. Who knows, you might just, very naturally, begin to strip your clothes off one night and seduce him as he has never been seduced before. Just remember the eye contact!

12

Hot Talk
and Whispers

I'm never dirty. I'm interesting without being vulgar.
I just...suggest.

—Mae West

"Ooh. Ahhhh. Ummm. Oh, baby..."

Many men really love when women communicate erotically with them in the bedroom and beyond. They like hot talk. A man wants to know he is giving you pleasure and he likes to keep count of your orgasms. Most importantly, he wants to be able to express himself freely and is far more comfortable doing so when you do it too!

If you are not used to communicating in the spirit of eroticism—in other words, hot talk—you may think you will sound dumb attempting to add some sizzle to your vocabulary.

Perhaps you think all erotic language is dirty, and the concept of talking dirty does not appeal to you or fit your style. Or maybe you are just one of those women who has "a mouth on her," yet can't get herself to utter any sizzling words or phrases of sexual acknowledgment to her lover. Part of the process of identifying your inner seductress and her seduction signature, is finding the hot talk that feels right for you and is stimulating for him; words and whispers of eroticism that are good for both of your souls.

You may do very well with some of the most traditional hot talk (you know, *those words,* the ones you can't say on TV!). And it is important to honor that and allow yourself to express it in whatever way is comfortable. There is no such thing as a dirty word; there are only dirty belief systems and negative attitudes about certain words that are, in another context, harmless. How about *pussy?* Pussy is a cat. And what about *cock.* A cock is a rooster. When you think of them as an apartment-dwelling pet and an early-rising farm bird, there's no charge in them. You can also take the charge out of them in bed because that's another place in which those words are harmless and, in fact, appropriate.

Maybe you need some flowery alternatives. Just keep in mind that the intention of hot talk is to steam things up, stimulate arousal, and keep the lines of communication open. The kinds of statements that will accomplish that are those that deliver the following messages:

- ♥ You are having a great time
- ♥ He is giving you great pleasure
- ♥ You want to give him great pleasure
- ♥ Isn't it great to share such great pleasure together
- ♥ You are so hot for him that you cannot control yourself
- ♥ He is such a great lover that you are in ecstasy
- ♥ You have never experienced such bliss
- ♥ You are still having a great time

- You, or one of you, is about to come…and you're happy about it
- You could do it all night because it feels so good

If you are one of those people who think erotic language will require confession at the end of the week or who fears you'll lose some karmic brownie points if you speak hot talk, then let it be. Speak in sweet nothings or heartfelt feelings.

However, if you are busting to say something wicked and wild, out loud, in bed, with your lover, then go for it. It may be a phrase as simple as: "Lover, you make me feel so good!" Or, for those of you who want to ride the edge of wilder erotic expression, it can be something like a blow-by-blow description of your orgasm process followed by the ever-popular "explosion": "Oh, Lover, I can feel myself beginning to pulsate with pleasure. Ah, it's beginning between my legs and spreading across my belly. I feel myself filling up. Oh…Oh…it feels so great…it's so tingly and wild…I'm…I'm…I'm coming."

It's all about sharing a little of your internal process, verbally, as you experience pleasure together. This keeps men very hot and engaged, because they know each sexual experience is more than just a stab in the dark. It's a communication orgy!

Test Your Hot-Talk Quotient

Although those who know me now would find it hard to believe, back in 1983 I was petrified—*petrified*—of saying erotic or "dirty" words out loud. I thought I sounded gross. I thought I was too much of a middle-class, white-bread girl to get away with it.

I dated a man who was a wonderful erotica writer and he used to read his work to me out loud. It was loaded with hot talk about female genitalia, the male organ, and what happens when you put the two together. One day he handed me an article and said, "You read." It would have been a great turn-on for him to hear me utter the words he'd written, but I couldn't bring myself to do it. I was scared silly. My stomach tightened, my throat got dry, my lips quivered.

"What's the matter," he asked. "They're just words, and it's just me sitting here listening. Read it for me...please."

Again, I froze. He let the incident slide, but I knew in my heart that I would not be happy if I allowed my fear of speaking certain words out loud to get in the way of experiencing pleasure. Because on the other side of my fear was a wild, erotic playground, the key to which were those secret passwords.

I made a mental list of all the four-letter words I couldn't utter in front of anyone, and I began to practice saying them. I'd say them around my cat. I'd say them to myself in the mirror. I would repeat each one ten times, every morning, until I began to gain more confidence.

Soon, the words for female organs that so horrified me became less frightening. The language to describe male anatomy, which seemed classier to begin with, became palatable. I started to slowly use them in lovemaking with the erotica writer. He was so generous and easygoing about hot talk that it became easy. Before I could say, "Forgive me, father, for I have sinned," we were spinning wild, erotic fantasies together, based on language. We acted out the priest and parishioner, the schoolgirl and the headmaster, the college professor and the student.

I learned how to say whatever I wanted to say without apologies. For me, it was a big thing.

Public Performances

One day, he began reading aloud to me from a new piece he'd written and, again, offered it to me to read. I said yes.

It was a start. A public reading for one, of someone else's words, was a little more risqué than talking to myself, and it began to help me expand my comfort level. Around the same time, I'd begun to write a sex novel, which was really beginning to loosen up my language about erotic anatomy. He'd go over the chapters with me while I read aloud. The language itself began to sound very neutral, like it was no big deal. The challenge was to find enough variations of words to describe the female and male anatomy so as not to be totally redundant!

Erotic Language Comes of Age

Of course, the big hoot is that years later, I went on to prove myself quite successful with erotic language. Not only did I launch a career in erotica writing, I taught courses on the topic and went on to become editor in chief of the nation's leading women's sex magazine.

I used dirty words all the time. By 1993 I had perfected the art of being a woman who could say anything in front of anyone. I reveled in my ability to make some men squirm with my comfort about sex. And I loved the freedom of sharing my intimate vocabulary with my intimate partners. My challenge became distinguishing what I could and couldn't say on TV while promoting my books (clitoris is fine, clit is not, for instance; erection was good, hard-on was not).

This helped me see that there is a real need in our culture for euphemisms for sexual organs and sexual acts. I started compiling a little dictionary of sex words, with the help of the students in my course, other sex writers, and people I worked with at *Playgirl* and Masquerade Books.

The first thing I did in all erotica classes was have people call out whatever word for female and male sexual parts came to mind. Everyone thinks they can handle it, until they have to say it out loud. And they think they know a lot of great words until they have to come up with a thousand different ways to say the same thing.

The first thing I did on my first day at *Playgirl* was challenge the staff to come up with ten words each for the female genitals, the male genitals, and the act of sexual intercourse.

If you are anxious to increase your comfort level with hot talk, yet concerned about whether you can pull it off, I suggest you try the same exercise, and try to find the right balance and tone of your personal approach to hot talk. In addition, use the following questions to assess your starting point and make some choices about how you would like to express your hot-talking seductress.

- Give five reasons why you want to talk hot talk
- Are there any dirty words that scare you? Why?
- Which words do you most want to incorporate into your personal hot talk vocabulary?
- Write down as many words as you can think of that describe female sexual parts
- Write down as many words as you can think of that describe male sexual parts
- Write down as many words and phrases as you can think of to describe the act of sexual intercourse
- Write down how sex with your man makes you feel
- Write down any nicknames you have or would like to bestow upon your lover and his love thing
- If you feel inhibited talking hot talk, can you put into words why?

An Erotic Vocabulary to Learn and Use

Just to give you a sense of how silly, and hot, language can be without being "dirty," take a look at some of the following compilations of my favorite words and those submitted by my *Playgirl* staff, my students, and from the *Pornographer's Dictionary,* a sex-word style sheet from the editors of Masquerade Books.

Penis

Love thing	John Thomas
Weenie	Willie
Charger	Wanker
Dick	Love bat
Love rod	Lingam
Spear	Little man
Hoo-haa	Small head
Rocket	Mr. Happy
Torpedo	Love sword
Baton	Sugar stick
Power tool	Moisture missile
Schlong	Trouser snake
Knob	Penetrator
Cow prod	Mighty missile
Sex serpent	Plumb head
Beef jerky	Prong
Shaft	Tallywhacker
Salami	Sex pistol
Poker	Love pistol

Vagina/Vulva/Clitoris

Love lips	Kitty lips
Cleopatra's clutch	She-petals
Sex-flesh	Honey pot
Gateway to Heaven	Love oven
(Love, Lust, etc.)	Little fox
Love canal	Love button
Female parts	Center
Down below	Opening
Honey	Love chasm
Passion cavern	Girl juice
Luscious lips	Netherlips

Sugar   Yoni
Twinkie   Love garden

Arousal

Pulsating   Creaming in my jeans
Hornier than an elk in   Hungry for your love
  rutting season   Open for you
In rut   Ready for you
Horny   In need of you
Hot for your body   Crazy for you
Throbbing for your thing   Desperate for your love
Anticipating your entry   Oh...*do me!*
Wet and wild for you

Sexual Intercourse and Play

Doing the wild thing   Push in the bush
Doing the nasty   The sexual shuffle
The horizontal bebop   Carnal cavort
In-and-out   Swaying the sheets
Humping   Horizontal mambo
Riding the waves   Boffing
Hiding the salami   Poking
Bobbing for beef   Sexperience
Home run

If you are one of those people who really wants to get down, with the most taboo language, it's time to start working it into your life. Practice with one or two words that you may have felt uncomfortable saying in the past, and just try using them when you're alone...in the shower, driving the car, washing dishes, masturbating. Include them in sentences and just say them out loud. Desensitizing yourself is a good place to start. Pick language that's going to have the strongest erotic charge—even if those are the words you're most nervous saying.

Once you begin to get a sense of the kind of language that is comfortable for you now, and the kind of stuff you'd like to work your way toward, practice...practice...practice! In no time, you'll be talking like a truck driver, or a hot-talking romantic—whichever is right for you.

To gauge your partner's response, look, listen, and hear his response. Don't ask him how he feels about what you're saying, or even what he thinks. See what his body does. If it talks back, then, I'd say you're on the right track!

13

Creating the Environment

There is a mood, setting, and energy for every type of seductive experience. Often the best way to create the mood for seduction is from the inside out: Tap into your inner seductress and then invite her out to play!

My friend Barbara Biziou, a teacher and expert on the art of creating rituals and author of a forthcoming book, *The Joy of Ritual* (Golden Books, 1998), says the best way to meet your inner seductress is to create the spirit of seduction and love around you and release her from within.

"We each have a sensual seductress living inside us, waiting to be released," says Biziou. "She is vibrant, confident, and totally in touch with her sexuality. She loves to touch and be caressed. She loves silk, warm bubble baths, fresh flowers, exotic scents. Put her in a room with sexy men and she's in heaven. Yet she is often ignored. I believe the challenge is that many women don't have a clue how to access her. In fact, many women are unaware that she even exists."

I asked Biziou to share a ritual of awakening, to help women access the inner sex goddess. She says you'll need the following items:

> Red candle
> Ylang-ylang and/or jasmine
> Papaya, banana, watermelon, clove
> Anything sweet (such as chocolate)
> Sensual music

Begin by turning off all the phones. Turn the lights down. Create a sensual atmosphere that will entice your inner seductress to come out. Light some of your favorite incense or place some essential oils in a diffuser (ylang-ylang, jasmine, and gardenia are some of the favored aphrodisiacs). Anoint yourself with your favorite perfume. Make sure that you dab some between your breasts and near your pubic bone. Lie with you knees up and open. Your feet are on the floor. Begin to take long deep breaths. Breathe in slowly to the count of four. As you breathe in, feel your abdomen expand. Feel the breath move into your pelvis. Place your hands over your pelvis and feel it expand with the in and out breath.

Now, begin to breathe in, as if the breath were coming through your vagina. These breaths will help connect you to the sensual, sexual woman inside. Let the breath flow like a river of energy. Feel the fluidity—the sensuality—and imagine that there is a passionate woman inside who wants to talk to you. Give her your inner ear and listen. See what she wants from you.

Notice: What kind of clothes does she wear? What does she like to eat? What makes her happy? What is her relationship with her body? How does she like to be touched? Take a few moments and allow her energy to infuse you. Remember, this is your imagination, so don't censor anything that comes forth. You don't have to edit. This is an exercise in free expression. Be open to receiving information that allows your innate sensuality to emerge.

Now slowly get up and run a warm bath. Put in some ylang-ylang or jasmine. (You can purchase these essential oils in a health food store.) Or pick any fragrance that makes you feel sensual and passionate.

Light a red candle (for passion), turn on some soft, sexy music, and melt into the fragrant water. Touch yourself as you would love to be touched.

After the bath, get into a bed made up with fresh, clean sheets—silk is great—and enjoy a feast of sensual delights. Let yourself feel and become the sensual woman you are inside; the woman you want to be! Dance naked and let your body move freely; feel the air against your naked flesh as you allow yourself to go with the flow. Let the sexy music lift you higher and higher as you get lost in the sensations of the moment. Allow the sensual, sexy, erotic being within to express herself. When you open your eyes, look in a mirror and you will see her…the Inner Seductress. Through elevating your own erotic energy level, you will bring her out!

If you need a little help in expressing yourself, Biziou suggests the following tonic to unleash the voluptuous instincts within. Mix together the following and sip slowly:

> One half cup papaya juice
> One quarter cup smashed banana
> One quarter cup watermelon juice
> One half teaspoon of powdered cloves

According to the delicious love video "Cupid's Arrow: The Secrets of Love Potions, Aphrodisiacs and Spells" (Central

Productions), Biziou's suggested tonic was the same one used by Cleopatra to put men of might into a passionate state. It was known as "Cleopatra's Elixir of Everlasting Love." Once a male sipped the Queen's sweet brew, he was her love slave. Biziou says that women can first empower themselves with the potions and scents they later share with their men. When it comes to many ancient tools of seduction, what's good for the goose is also good for the gander!

The Queen of the Nile also soaked the sails of her barges in jasmine, so that men could pick up her scent from miles away as she traveled on the river. The scent created a stimulus response: passion, arousal, and excitement. When a woman bathes herself in the scent, she is igniting the possibility of passion within herself and honoring her own erotic impulses. But who knows what will happen if her man gets a whiff or a sniff—aphrodisiac scents, along with a woman's unleashed expression of her inner goddess, are a very powerful combination! A woman does not have to go wild in front of a man; it's a very private moment of self-expression. Yet the act of unleashing the sensual woman within will automatically impact her sensual communication with a man!

Biziou suggests that if Cleopatra's love potion is not available or not tasty for you, you might prefer the following mixture as an alternative sensual brew:

> A glass of cool milk
> spiced with cinnamon
> a dash of rose water

If that elixir isn't available or palatable, try a cup of hot chocolate, a drink of grape juice or, the old standby, a glass of wine.

Biziou advises you to really enjoy the taste sensations as they slide down your throat. Feel the coolness or the warmth, the slight sting of citrus or the soft flow of grape. Experience the sipping of the potion as part of the sensual moment. Keep on dancing, and inviting your inner seductress onto the dance floor of your erotic expression. Then fantasize, fantasize, fantasize. Everything that occurs in life begins as a thought, a wish, a vision, a dream. By evoking the sensual seductress within through your own self-love ritual, you are creating the environment and setting the mood for inviting in your sensual spirit of love and seduction.

I encourage you to play and have fun, experiment, and take risks...and stay true to yourself and your desires! Repeat the ritual for accessing the seductress within as often as needed. It is a private meditation available to you at any time!

Aural Sex

A good story can make marvelous things happen. It stirs the soul, and touches the heart, and will encourage your inner seductress to emerge. Play it while alone, and while with your lover.

Erotica, from Love Story Classics, is the audiotape every woman should pop in the cassette player just before a sex date or while on a sensual self-love date. The deep, sultry voice of narrator J. P. Linton especially stirs you with the promise of hot things to come. His cultured reading of several steamy classics, including "Love In Athens," by Frank Harris and "Once," by D. H. Lawrence, go straight from the ears to the clitoris, steeping you in anticipation. By the time your beloved arrives, you will be wet and wild with desire! And if no date looms on the horizon, the audio can serve as the impetus for a self-love ritual of elegant lust! (Order from Love Story Classics, P.O. Box 1952, New York, NY 10113.)

Music can also make marvelous things happen. Set the mood with the right romantic music. Essex Entertainment has a series of Romantic Classics CDs that appeal to all sensual appetites. Start your evening with *Seduction,* a captivating collection of Mozart masterpieces. Do dinner to *Passion,* a Tchaikovsky treasure of tunes that gets blood rushing to all the right places. *Ecstasy,* with its softly intense collection by masters of romance, is perfect for making out. *Rapture,* with it's scintillating, soaring melodies, will magnify the pleasures of lovemaking. Cool down and bask in the afterglow with *Intimacy.* Each CD empowers a different stage of loving. If you are planning a quickie, try one CD; for a full evening of love, try all—they run over an hour each. These are available in most CD stores.

For the journey from foreplay to intercourse, and then to help you chill out after the loving, try *Music for Lovemaking.* Conceived by musician Douglas Berlent, the music evokes passion and inspires consummation in slow, orchestrated stages. This CD turns sex into a delicious eight-course meal, rather than a fast-food quickie. For instance, the Tango and Bolero-like "Tangelero" gets the juices flowing, whether you are vertical or horizontal. "The Man" and "The Woman" celebrate the energy of both sexes. And "The Kiss" brings you to that moment of slobbering all over each other like primates in heat just before his arrow finds its way to your core! By the time you hear "Harmonic Ocean" and "Primal Chant," your sexual motors will be on overdrive. Then, there's "Afterglow."

Music For Lovemaking II, also conceived by Doug Berlent, was developed at an Ivy League university by some really smart musicians who know that good music inspires great sex! This is music that makes you hot, inspires you to do it, and provides a great backdrop for sensuality and romance. The music—from Spain, Brazil, France, Italy, Africa, and Argentina—includes biofeedback generated sound-scapes that seem to penetrate the soul! (Order both CDs from Media Right Music, 324 W. 23rd St., Ste. 3-B, New York, NY 10011.)

If you're temporarily singing the boredom in the bedroom blues, Steven Halpern's *Enhancing Sensual Pleasure* can jump-start a sleepy love life. This "Subliminal Soundtrack for

Consenting Adults" delivers sex-positive messages that will pump up the passion, such as "You turn me on" and "I love the way you touch me." You don't actually "hear" them, but your subconscious, and your partner's, will. Positive sex statements are delivered beneath the sexy, sensual sound of Halpern's soothing new-age type music—all tingly tunes perfect for dancing the horizontal tango. A sure thing for self-lovers, as well. (Order from Xandria Collection, P.O. Box 319005, San Francisco, CA 94134.)

Feng Shui

There are many subtle secrets for creating an environment of allure and arousal that have been around for eons. The ancient practice of Feng Shui (pronounced *fung shway*), which has gained wide popularity lately, is one of them.

Feng Shui focuses on how people experience the places they inhabit or visit. The art originated thousands of years ago in China, yet the principles are applicable in any culture—even in the boudoir, or anywhere else you plan to seduce your intended.

As Feng Shui master Nancilee Wydra explains it, "Harmonious living spaces can add measurably to life's satisfactions and that premise is at the heart of feng shui. Feng Shui identifies conditions in our living space that affect us in either positive or negative ways." She goes on to say: "According to Feng Shui, the language of an environment tells a story, and if we change the elements of our surroundings, we can improve the story. We can orchestrate our fate by manipulating an environment."

While Feng Shui is used in homes, offices, and many innovative health and healing centers, it can also be used to set the stage for a successful seduction—one in which the elements are placed to favor love and passion.

Wydra, a consultant, columnist, and author of numerous books on the topic, including *Feng Shui: Book of Cures; Designing Your Happiness;* and *Feng Shui for Singles,* says Feng Shui can be conducive to great allure and loving and offers very simple and practical tips for creating an environment of seduction in your home. "You have to set the stage, and do things that are subliminal," she says. "Your home, and every choice you make, reflects you in ways that you don't even know."

Begin to set the seduction stage at your doorway, for it is the entrance to your world, and it is in that entrance that your beloved, or intended beloved, should have his very first experience of you. Wydra offers some practical tips that she uses in her Feng Shui practice and courses.

Scent

"Use a scent at the door," Wydra suggests. There are many to choose from. Visit a health food store and choose from a wide selection of essential oils and scented candles, each meant to accomplish different things. Wydra offers the following suggestions:

- If your lover is a type A kind of person, use spiced apple scent at the door. It will give the sense of immediate spiciness and uplifting possibilities.
- If your man is there for a first date, or it is a relatively new relationship, use mint. It will relax and calm him. It will erase nervousness and help him enter with a clear mind—rather than the kind of imaginings that first date jitters and new love sometimes inspire!

Lighting

The mistake that most of us make is trying to create dimness or darkness around ourselves and keeping light away. It is a myth that darkness is sexy. If we don't make the "edge" of the light in the environment clear, this takes the edge off of seduction in a nanosecond.

"Make sure your lighting is low on the outside of your immediate area, and brighter on you," she says. "If you have a light on in the bathroom, the hallway, the vestibule, or outside the bedroom, it kills the edge. The lighting behind the couch or behind the chair must be dimmer, not lighter."

When the lighting is not in proper perspective, she says, the seductress tends to look, well...terrible. Although women tend to think low lights means a multitude of sins are being hidden, according to Feng Shui, that's not true.

"If you don't feel comfortable about your body, and you know you are going to be naked, get a moving light," she suggests. The movement helps to diffuse and soften the contours of the body and give us a sense of freedom because it is moving.

She suggests buying a mirrored disco ball (à la *Saturday Night Fever*, but smaller) or putting a fan in front of a lamp. Each creates the sense of moving light, which is just what the Feng Shui master orders for women who feel uncomfortable in their own flesh and yet want to enhance their confidence and seductive powers. "Anything that will create a shadow and give the effect of light twirling around the room will help," she says.

Another trick is to position a special spotlight in the seduction area and dangle a multifaceted, clear crystal (it can be smaller than a golf ball) in front of it at a distance that allows the light to bounce off the crystal and dance around the room. The crystal has the added advantage of having a healing effect. It makes the room, you, and your man feel healthier.

Candles

Candles are a welcome addition to any seduction, yet Wydra points out, "If candlelight is on your face, you're going to look disgusting."

The seductress who utilizes Feng Shui sex tips should find a safe and appropriate way to keep the flicker of candlelight off her face, preferably by placing it above her head. "The candle should be higher up than you are—on a shelf, for instance, not on the night table—or it should be a bigger, taller, higher candle or candlestick."

Flowers

Roses are always an inspiring sight and fragrance for women, and they can support an evening of seduction by sending off a sweet scent and looking pretty.

"Roses strengthen the sense of self," Wydra points out. "That's why when you receive roses they make you feel good about yourself." She says that women typically do not feel empowered enough, which is why they love roses.

Wydra cautions that the only time you want to stay clear of roses is if your beloved or intended is someone who is overly enthusiastic about himself. "No roses for the egomaniac," she says. "They will empower him too much!"

Colors

There are a number of colors that enforce seductive feelings, such as red—the color of passion—yet some colors will take the wind right out of the chimes of a good seduction.

"If your bedroom is green or yellow, you might want to throw something over the bedspread or change the sheet to another color," she points out. "This is because few of us look good surrounded by or on top of the colors yellow and green."

You don't have to redecorate your environment, just tone down those colors if they happen to be yours!

If you are open to redecorating for seductress success, try a red bedspread and sheets on for size. If it's softer, more sacred communion you seek, use soft blue to indigo and lavender.

A Soft, Sensual Touch

The sense of touch and thermal comfort is of the utmost importance in seduction, and Wydra says women should assess their living space, or designated seduction area, for anything that may be rough, abrasive, or unpleasant against naked flesh. Do this before the big night!

"Walk around the house naked, sit on things, or place yourself against things. If it's scratchy against your tush, then it's not good," she points out.

"If your sofa is wool or some other scratchy material, then you should toss a Chanel silk or tapestry over it...one that's silky, soft, or satiny. That kind of material is inviting and welcoming. Harsh fabrics push people away and repel your seductive efforts."

Although there are many ways to create an environment conducive to seduction, the Feng Shui approach is quickly gaining recognition as a practice that can literally change one's entire life. Feng Shui can alter the look of your home, but more important, can alter the experience you have there, the experience your lover has there, and the experience you share together.

14

Toys "R" Us

The first key to being a great seductress is the ability to be one's own lover.

One of the most important tenets of sexual expression is: Don't be afraid to touch yourself and be responsible for your own pleasure. A woman who knows the erotic nuances of her own body is a seductress supreme. Not only does she demonstrate an openness to her own body, she lets a guy off the hook and helps him feel that he has a partner in passion, rather than a woman waiting passively to be pleased!

What turns you on and what pleases you most is often found at the touch of your own hands. One of the most popular ways to explore self-pleasuring through masturbation is by using what was once known as a personal massager or a marital aid. These days, a vibrator can be a girl's best friend. Many women find that incorporating sex toys into their boudoir routine, or using a sex toy to masturbate for a man, is an extraordinary turn-on.

The art of inserting something penislike into the vagina and pumping to simulate sexual intercourse is almost as ancient as sex itself. According to *Sex Facts: The Handbook for the Carnally Curious* (Citadel Press, 1992), the ladies (and sometimes men) of yore used dildoes made of leather, sometimes in sexual performances or exhibitions. The device was known as an olisboi, which means "to glide or slip."

Sex Toys Come of Age

There was a time, not so long ago, that sex toys were taboo. Not anymore! The sex-toy industry is now a huge, multimillion-dollar industry spawned by the age of latex and the desire of couples to add a little pizzazz into their lovemaking. The selection of sexy playthings and accessories is beyond imagination. Have you tried the Lovers' Swing? Do you know about the video that demonstrates how to free the female orgasm? Are you aware of the him-and-her love toys designed to titillate you both to ecstasy?

These are the toys that mom never told you about—and they are not your mother's vibrator. Hers—if she dared have one—was likely a rocket-ship shaped item molded in hard plastic that made a loud buzz; she probably purchased it on a lark in a Times Square drugstore while wearing a big hat and dark sunglasses. Today, there are a multitude of cute and classy sex boutiques, such as Eve's Garden in New York and Good Vibrations in San Francisco, or you can order toys by mail (see listings on page 138).

There are a wild array of sexual goodies that can be used in a safe and healthy way. Latex love-things, G spot stimulators, and sex enhancers for him and her come in all shapes, sizes, colors, and textures. They wiggle, squiggle, vibrate, probe, plunge, and bring you to ecstasy. Playful and slightly kinky, there is a bounty of pleasure toys, games, novelty items, films, and sexy books that will ignite your imagination. Sex toys can expand your sexual horizons and pleasure.

It's important to note that using a sex toy should no longer be an embarrassment. There is a toy for every occasion and one appropriate for every woman, man, or couple. While the old attitude about sex aids may have been that couples who used them were people on the fringes of life, and women who owned vibrators were desperate for a man or suffering from nymphomania, the new attitude is that couples who use them are capable of deeper intimacy and more expansive sexuality, and a woman who plays solo is a woman in charge of her own pleasure!

Used and cleaned properly, many of the toys on the market today are healthy and can be great fun in bed! These toys will help you expand your sexual repertoire, teach you where all your pleasure spots are, and help train you to be a better lover. They can also help you locate your man's hot spots. Many men hate the burden of making things happen in bed, or they are afraid they are not giving a woman what she wants. Men appreciate a lover who knows how to pleasure herself and can show a man—in nonthreatening ways—how to please her.

Love toys can enhance your seductive abilities in the bedroom because they:

- expand sexual consciousness and open the door to new sexual adventures
- add a dimension of experimentation and newness that can fuel the fires of passion
- take the pressure off the male partner, because he knows he can ensure his woman's orgasm, regardless of the strength of his erection
- give the woman the opportunity to learn what most pleases her, and then show her partner how by guiding him to the right spots
- can physically enable you to reach spots in the male and female anatomy that are sometimes difficult to locate or maintain contact with using fingers, such as the prostate in the man or the G spot in the woman

Self-Love

Before you experiment with sex toys, make sure you set aside some alone time. My recommendations for a good self-pleasure ritual are:

1. Be sure you will have undisturbed time alone. The kids and hubby should be out, or safely tucked away in another part of the house, so you don't have to worry about them walking in or hearing you call out. It shouldn't be the day the cleaning lady will be there or the workmen are fixing windows. Give yourself time without distractions.
2. Treat yourself like a lover. If you were treating a guest to a sexy session of love, how would you set the mood? Flowers? Pretty scents? A warm bath before and a soft nap after? Give to yourself what you would give to a lover.
3. Enjoy audiovisual stimulation. There's nothing wrong with listening to a hot audiotape or watching an erotic video—either a movie or a "training film." Women are a growing segment of the consumers of erotic films. It is often women who account for the majority of X-rated video rentals.
4. Feel free to have an orgasm derby. When I watched Candida Royalle's *The Gift* I challenged myself to have an orgasm with every hot sex scene (there are many). After the film was over, I had experienced six orgasms. It reminded me of the old days, when I had all the time in the world to pleasure myself.

Sex Toys for Self-Pleasure

I believe in creating rituals for self-pleasure. It's something I learned to do as a sex toy reviewer for *Playgirl*, where I had the opportunity to test-drive many new products and rate them for readers. I would pull down the shades, take the phone off the hook, dim the lights, and spend an afternoon alone in bed, reveling in the experience of self-pleasuring and experimentation.

To set the mood, I would often light a candle and pop a sensual CD or video on. I would take a warm scented bath or spend some time touching myself in a way that I would want a lover to touch me. I got quite adept at the art of self-pleasure by going through this process at least once a month. As you can imagine, it was one of the best jobs I've ever had. I got paid for having pleasure.

But even when I wasn't "working," the ritual of self-love was a wonderful way to give to myself and to really learn how I liked to be touched and where. It made me a better lover and a better communicator. Knowing my own pleasure spots gave me more confidence and I found that sharing them with a man was a real turn-on for us both.

How to Introduce Sex Toys

If you decide to bring playthings to your passion play, make it fun. Nothing is less seductive than introducing a love toy as if you are about to start a serious science project. Now, a fun science project, that's something different. If playing with love toys is a virgin voyage for you, treat it that way, and go about experimenting with all the awe of a teenager just learning how to have sex. While most devices come with instructions on the box and are easy to use, a newcomer may feel slightly clumsy at first. Don't fret. Remember, it's supposed to be a sex *toy,* not a sex stifler!

Getting used to sexy playthings may take practice, and you may find it's not for you—or your man. When you intend to introduce a toy to a lover, set the mood in a way that you know will be conducive to his participation. It could be the softly erotic atmosphere you give to yourself during self-pleasure, or something slightly wilder, depending on the guy. The idea is to make it safe—safe for him to open up and experiment with you—and fun.

Select a toy or device you feel would be acceptable to him. Perhaps he would enjoy a French tickler (a nonvibrating device that goes over the penis, or on it, and stimulates the woman) or maybe he would enjoy a toy that penetrates the anus and touches what is called the male sacred spot in Tantric sexuality. Massaging of that spot can give pleasure and healing to a man. Obviously, if you sense he would hate having that part of his body touched, don't get a sex toy designed to touch that part. Try something else.

Susan Crain Bakos, author of *Sexational Secrets: Exotic Advice Your Mother Never Told You* (St. Martin's Press, 1996), once told me that there were two things she considered key to great sex. "A woman should always take responsibility for herself," she said, "and a finger up the anus never hurts."

I share this to suggest that you may have to initiate your man to anal play by way of utilizing your fingers, but that doesn't preclude the possibility he will some day be interested in a sex toy designed to do the same!

Which Toys Are for You?

The marketplace is full of fantastic devices designed to enhance sexual pleasure. All you need is a couple of batteries (if even) and a sense of fun to find the right toy for you and your mate.

Vibrators these days come in all shapes and sizes, practically tailor-made to the shape of any individual woman's vagina, and packed with varying degrees of power. While the standard hard plastic vibrator is still used by some, it has spawned an entirely new generation of toys that tremble and throb within the inner sanctum of a woman. Some are soft latex and jellylike. Some are shaped like animals and even have a smaller attachment designed to stimulate the clitoris while the larger one is stirring inside the woman. There are even vibrators that strap around the legs and can be placed right on the clitoris offering delightful direct stimulation; these can be used separately or in conjunction with penile penetration! Vibrators built to fit in the vagina can also be used to stimulate the nipples—of both partners.

Some "vibrators" don't vibrate—they are simply latex love toys of varying shapes and sizes. You can almost certainly find one that will fill the vagina with the same depth and width of a mate's penis; or even discover one that is shaped specifically for intense contact with the G spot. These items range from lifelike latex or rubber penises, molded to actually have veins on the surface and a base of rubber testicles, to small, smooth, slightly curved latex items that are smooth or even psychedelic-looking on the surface.

There is an entire industry built on toys to titillate the anus alone, including everything from what is commonly known as a "butt plug" to slim and vibrating penetrative devices.

If it turns out that you are not a Sex Toys "R" Us kid, remember: These items are always a great conversation piece. Just buying one and suggesting its use will expand your sexual confidence and open the lines of sexual communication between you and the man you aim to seduce.

Sex Toy Picks

Just to get you started, here are my recommendations. These are all toys that are fun, pleasurable and easy to order. Many of them can be ordered from one of the following three popular sources:

- ❤ Good Vibrations, 938 Howard Street, Suite 101, San Francisco, CA 94103
- ❤ Nasstoys, 20–40 Jay Street, Brooklyn, New York, NY 11201
- ❤ Stamford Hygienic, P.O. Box 1160, Long Island City, NY 11101

For Going Solo

Get Some Good Loving From a Pisces Pisces men are usually very creative lovers, and the Pisces Pearl follows suit. It's a translucent green, vibrating, rubberized penis that has a soft clitoral stimulator shaped like a fish. It's the size of an average man with a smooth, circumcised head that features a mustached face (this is because it's made in Japan, where the law says that sex toys have to look like people, animals, or fish). Like a fish, the surface feels slightly slimy—so give it a good cleansing before insertion, or use a condom. I know it sounds bizarre-looking, but it is one of the most delightful sex toys I've ever tried.

Before even installing batteries, try some lubricant and get used to inserting the toy and trying some simple thrusting movements until the back-and-forth sloshing movement inspires you to plunge more aggressively. At the same time, you can press the little fish against your clitoris, or gently bend it out of the way. When you finally put Mr. Pisces in vibrating mode, the pearls—stashed gumball-machine-style in the center—vibrate and tumble at the rim of the vagina, stimulating some some of the most super-sensitive nerve endings in your body. Meanwhile, Mr. Pisces's entire penile body vibrates and undulates at many different speeds, setting off a collaboration of explosive tinglies. The real kicker is the way the fish simultaneously vibrates on the clitoris (also at varying speeds, which you control).

Batteries are inserted at the base of this toy, but, if a hot-pink phallus with a bunny and battery attachment is more your style, try the Rabbit Pearl, which has the same scintillating effects. Order from Good Vibrations.

Works Like Magic   Every girl should have her very own Flex-a-Pleaser. It's a vibrating "wiggle stick" that works like a magic wand, capable of satisfying any need! The device looks like a small golf club; yet the flexible, bendible shaft ends in a slim, round-tip vibrator that incites a titillating "tee-off." In fact, this nifty nightstick can tickle, tease, and slide into any "hole" on your body, or a friend's! It's also a great device for tantalizing your favorite external erogenous zones—nipples, clitoris, the head of his "iron"!

The easy-to-grasp, multispeed power handle is equipped with an easy-to-work sliding lever that zooms from mild vibrations to high-speed stimulation in a flash! All you need is a couple of AA batteries and you're on your way to nirvana. Order from Stanford Hygienic.

The Water Toy You Can Take Anywhere   Every woman should have at least one water toy—and I don't mean a rubber ducky. The Wet and Dry Aquassager is a versatile little vibrator that fits in a pocket and can be used in a bathtub, pool, or lake— or on dry land. At six inches long and less then two inches in diameter, it has the advantage of being compact and portable. It's got a relatively low hum, so it's easy to use, discreetly, anywhere (I've tried it personally on a plane and in a movie theater bathroom, just to see how discreet it is!); when immersed in water, it's completely inaudible. When you are sitting in the bath and enjoying the feel of warm water swooshing between your lower parts, the Aquassager will finish the job. Just know it could take a spell: While the device packs a surprising amount of power for such a small, one-battery device, it has one speed, so it's all in the way you operate it.

The Aquassager comes with three attachments that can be used for clitoral stimulation and other practical purposes: heel-shaped (for massage of the labia and foot rubs); coin-shaped (for slightly pressuring the clitoris and for facials); and gumdrop-shaped (for electronic kisses of the clitoris and pressure point massages to the shoulder). You can even stimulate your sex flesh with the smooth, removable cover. Order from Good Vibrations.

For Couples

It'll Rub You the Right Way   Once you figure out how to use the Sensual Lovers Ring, it will provide a delightfully different pleasure for you and your man. At first glance, it looks too funny to be a serious sex toy; and the average guy might find it just a tad intimidating. It is a ring with pleasure dots attached to an egg that is covered with ticklers, and it's supposed to be slipped over your man's manhood.

Ah, but once you slip it around his hot rod, and he slips it to you, you're heaven bound! Here's how it works: Slide the erect penis through the center of the ring; the tickler covered egg-shaped vibrator should be on the underside of his penis, so that when he penetrates you, the egg is right above your labia and clitoris. It takes some getting used too, but you and your honey can get into a rhythm that vibrates you both to orgasm!

The ring has tiny, flexible flaps that open to allow his penis through, and then give it a snug hug as it vibrates. The multiple-speed, nubbly tickler works the woman with sensual and exciting vibrations that pack a wallop. It takes two AA batteries. Order from Stamford Hygienic Corporation.

"Look At Us...We're Flying"   Gymnastics in the bedroom will never be the same after the Lovers Swing. This thick, sturdy, foam-filled braid covered with velvet comes alone, or with two love handles, to support your arms. You're set for deliciously deep sex as soon as you get the swing suspended over your bed—with lag bolts (hardware included)—or looped over the pricey Lover's Gym. Installation can be a challenge—unless you've got a darn sturdy ceiling and the ability to use a drill, hammer, and screwdriver—yet using the swing is like having sex in space: effortless and weight-free (it holds up to 300 lbs!). Float over your lover's penis, or face, rocking back and forth with just the right motion and merge your sexflesh with your man's in a deliciously magical way. It frees your hands to caress his flesh, instead having to hold yourself up for balance. Order from Body & Soul Productions, 5257 River Rd., Ste. 200, Bethesda, MD 20815-1415.

Splish-Splash in a Vibrating Bath   If you already think sharing a bath with your honey is a hot, intimate time, take the

ShowTime Waterproof Brush Massager with you to the next tub date! Not only is it a pure pleasure to scrub-a-dub your lover with deliciously vibrating bristles, it has a second attachment (smooth plastic with tiny vibrating nubs) that will send you into orgasmic spasms if placed strategically against the clitoris or over the entire mons. For a really fun time, soap and clean your lover's entire body with the slightly scratchy bristles; and let him do the same for you. Then switch to the smooth nubs, begin with the feet, calves, up between the thighs (ooh, ooh, ooh), and then smack between the legs. If direct vibration from attachments doesn't work for you, pressing the smooth, slightly nubby handle against your clitoris will probably put you over the top! And, just watch what happens when you place it on the underside of his testicles! There will be a lot of splashing for joy with this toy. Order from Good Vibrations.

"Ooooh, It Feels So Real!" Thanks to a nifty little invention called the Fleshlight, you'll never have to send your honey to bed hungry again.

The Fleshlight is a penis-friendly sex toy that you can use on your partner, or give him as a gift. It's shaped like a fat flashlight on the outside; inside is a simulated vagina that welcomes Mr. Happy with a warm, mushy, slishy sex feel. With the help of lubrication, the deliciously soft material grips and slips over your man like a glove and is deep enough to accommodate up to nine inches of his pulsating passion.

Here's how it works: Remove the caps on either end, slip out the plastic love lips insert, place it in warm or hot tap water for about five seconds, towel dry, slip it back into the casing, and lubricate liberally. Lubricate him liberally, as well, and slip his tip into the opening; watch his woody swell within the soft embrace of the womanlike toy. Simulating a woman-on-top position, press down while he presses in. The rest is like intercourse—and you know how to do that! After he comes, wash her up, pat her dry, and store her for future use. Fleshlight was invented by Steve Shubin, a former California cop and father of five who has derived much pleasure from testing the product with the help of his wife, a former tennis pro. Aside from being devoted to promoting the device as a safe sex toy, and a vehicle for sexual fulfillment for people with disabilities, Shubin says it's a great combatant of "not-tonight-honey-blues." Just for fun, Fleshlight comes in an assortment of colors—from fleshlike pink to bright blue and midnight black. In addition to the very detailed female model it's available in a mold made of a simple slit and a mold made in the image of deliciously pouty lips. Order from Interactive Life Forms, P.O. Box 141935, Austin, TX, 78714.

Better Than Strip Poker   "Think of yourself as a gift of food. Offer your partner a 'sample of you' that will taste wonderful." That's just one of the delicious instructions in Romantic Sensations, a lovers' game that offers an experience filled with sensual exploration and adventure. The game comes with Sensual Bath Gel and Sensuous Massage Lotion, so you'll be somewhat prepared to act on the impromptu suggestions. In the process of picking out cards in the categories of touch, taste, scent, and sound, you and your playmate can delve into each other's passions and pleasure with uninhibited spontaneity. The cards, which have quotes from famous people, as well as directions, challenge all your senses! How can you resist a dare such as this: "Tell your partner about an activity that you haven't done together before that you'd like to share with him, now!" Order from Games Partnerships Ltd., Inc, 116 New Montgomery, Ste. 500, San Francisco, CA 94105.

The Doctor Is In...on CD-ROM   For those too shy, or too cheap, to consult a sex therapist, Ann Hooper's Ultimate Sex Guide is now available on an enlightening and entertaining CD-ROM. Dr. Hooper, a charming Brit who dispenses advice on all manner of sexual curiosities and challenges, anticipates your every question with a vast "Sexopedia" containing files on a myriad of sexual situations—from ancient secrets of the Kama Sutra to modern sex games and toys.

While the doctor (who has a book by the same name) dispenses no-nonsense advice in a very user-friendly manner, the presentation on CD-ROM does have that Max Headroom-like quality to it, as Hooper appears regularly, a talking head, to guide people along.

In addition to the "Sexopedia," the CD-ROM has three other key components: "Questionnaires," which are the user's private files; "Programs for Better Sex," recommended therapeutic programs; and "Case Files," which profile other people's problems and how they solved them.

A fascinating interactive capability allows you to have an actual computer therapy session, plus, you'll find some sexy video demonstrations for your viewing pleasure. To order by mail write to: Order Processing, Houghton Mifflin, Wayside Rd., Burlington, MA 01803.

Hypnotic and Erotic   If your sex life is sagging and needs a jump-start, or if you really want to give yourself permission to live out some of your wildest fantasies, try psychologist Kevin Grold's Hypnosex program, which promises sexual ecstasy through self-hypnosis. It's not a masturbation series; instead, you relax and let your subconscious mind do all the work. The seven-week program is designed to free your imagination, move you past barriers, unlock your sexual spirit and set it free in the bedroom. It's Grold's voice that leads you through visualization exercises such as envisioning your most delicious fantasy playing on a VCR. He reminds you of a time when you were playful, uninhibited, free.

Repetition is the key as every week builds on the next. You listen to the same tape for at least five days, for about twenty minutes, beginning with a warm-up hypnosis exercise that links pleasure to your PC (pubococcygeus) muscles—just squeeze, anytime and anyplace, and you're filled with positive sexual feelings. By the time the program comes to an end, sexual experiences should be more intense, fulfilling, and freeing. Order from Life Publications, 2923 Camino Del Mar, Ste. 6, Del Mar, CA 90214-2052.

A Road Map to Your G Spot   Still searching for that elusive internal sexflesh? If you're ready to discover the legendary source of five-star orgasms, and learn to come beyond your wildest imaginings, get How to Female Ejaculate. This tape helps redefine the clitoris, show it's connected to the G spot, and detail how women can have mind-blowing ecstasy—and ejaculations that shoot clear across a room! As the narrator, Fanny Fatale, points out, explaining her first: "It was one of those slow, delicious orgasms that start in your toes, spread through your body, and explode in a burst of emotional and physical release, only this time it was accompanied by a big gush of liquid."

The video is two-thirds anatomy lesson: First, an explanation of female sexual physiology and video view of an actual G spot. And then, a casual chat between women enthusiasts of intense orgasmic pleasure! It wraps with a sizzling hot, very hands-on demonstration of four women coming, and coming again, in a titillating circle-jerk. Just join in! Order from Stamford Hygienic.

15

Your Body's Secret Weapon

A benefit of exploring the arena of sex toys is that it can help you become more conscious of strengthening one of the most important muscles in your body—the pubococcygeus muscle, affectionately known as the "love muscle." It's located in the pelvic floor—the gateway to the vagina. Some people call it "Cleopatra's Clutch," because this muscle has been the seductress's secret weapon for keeping men under her spell. A woman who controls that muscle well can look forward to enhanced pleasure and health—and a deeper connection to her man, who will feel more deeply accepted and taken in by his woman.

The pubococcygeus, or PC muscle, is a pelvic sling that extends from the front—the pubic bone—to the rear—the coccyx. It's present in both men and women.

God made the PC muscle to control the flow of urine—and to help a woman get a good grip on a man's penis. The muscle will clutch and clench around the penis (or anything that penetrates the vagina). It is the muscle that often twitches involuntarily when a man penetrates a woman, giving him great pleasure as well—sometimes causing him to orgasm before he really wants to. When it's toned and strong, a woman has greater control over when she does and doesn't clutch, and she has more intense orgasms. By doing Kegel exercises, a woman can make the vaginal ring become tighter, which gives her a better grip on her man.

The love muscle rules because it allows a woman to grasp a man and pull him deep inside, hold him, or drive him wild with the clasping caress of her muscles closing on his organ. The by-product of a woman's active utilization of her clutch comes with great perks—it enhances her pleasure, make her orgasms strong, and keeps her sexual area healthy.

Since this muscle can weaken as time marches on, one way to test it (for women and men) is to try to stop the flow of urine midstream. When the muscles are weak, it's difficult to just cut off the flow, indicating that the weakened PC muscles can thus become a health and hygiene issue; when the muscle is stronger, there is more control.

Kegels

Kegel exercises were named after Dr. Arnold Kegel, who discovered that exercising the PC muscles helped women who had urinary stress incontinence. Tightening the PC muscles lifts and strengthens the entire area. As many women learn in their childbearing years, Kegels are strongly recommended by doctors to strengthen and tone that essential muscle in the vagina both before the birth of a child, to prepare the pelvic floor for the trauma of birth, and immediately after the birth, when that part of a woman's body is weakest. Kegels are the best and most proven way to bring speedy healing to the area and regain strength, tone, and elasticity.

Do Your Kegels, Girls!

Kegels are simply the act of exercising the PC muscle by opening and closing the vagina with a clenching motion— the way one might stretch and then relax a rubber band between two fingers. It is always recommended that women do a rapid succession of these motions, such as ten sets of ten, ten times a day. They can be done anywhere—while driving, or standing on a supermarket line.

The Kegelcisor assists this by giving the PC muscle something to grasp, and training it to grasp harder and stronger by increasing the size of the "barbells" (the rounded knobs that graduate in size as the device moves further into the vagina). The added dimension of using the Kegelcisor is that is feels great, can make practice and training loads of fun, and enhances female sexual physiology in many ways. Besides, practicing the Kegels in bed is the most delightful way to get your exercise done, any day!

"The enhanced benefit to a woman is better sexual health," says sex therapist Richard Cohn. "The sexual perk for a couple is that lovemaking can be heightened for both parties. Kegel exercises circulate more blood to the sexual area; they help increase a feeling of awareness in the genitals and increase sexual arousal. When women practice regularly it creates a feeling of tightness, gives better friction during intercourse, and can also increase the movement of the clitoral hood, heightening arousal."

Making Exercise Fun!

One of the disappointments couples face as they age is that the vagina can become no longer tight enough to create desirable pressure and "hold" on the penis.

A "Kegelcisor" is like a tiny barbell designed for the vagina.

Not only does it feel delicious inside a woman, it gives her a sense of power and control over her female anatomy. The Kegelcisor is to the vagina what gym equipment is to the other muscles of the body. A woman can practice Kegel without this device; however, just as gym equipment helps strengthen your biceps, the Kegelcisor helps train the pubococcygeus muscle. Taking a Kegelcisor into the bedroom is also a perfect way for a couple to discover a healthy pleasure, together. (It can be ordered through Stamford Hygienic or Good Vibrations, listed in chapter 15.)

Kegels for Men

A man can also exercise his PC muscle, and Kegels have perks for him too. They can help him improve sexual function, attain stronger erections, and develop more genital sensitivity. A man's PC muscle is also located in the pelvic floor. Just as for a woman, it is the muscle that allows him to stop and control the flow of urine and can also raise and lower the penis.

It is more fun to try the exercises with the help of his seductress. While the penis is in the vagina, your guy can "exercise" by squeezing the muscle and allowing it to move up and down inside his woman. You know it's the PC muscle when you feel the penis move upward, often reaching the top of a woman's womb and touching her G spot in the process.

Lovers can play a delightful game of "dueling PC muscles," where each partner clenches and squeezes their sex muscle simultaneously. You can try it a couple of ways:

- During intercourse, when the penis is deep inside the vagina, the man can squeeze his PC muscles and the woman can follow each of his movements with her own squeeze! This is a fun— really fun—way to test the strength of the PCs.
- If you're really up for an adventure, have your man place his penis at the front of your vagina, right at the vaginal ring, and

slowly squeeze upward, as you squeeze and attempt to pull the penis in with the clutch of your PC muscle.

These exercises can be delightful and pleasurable for both of you. The squeezing motion as well as the movement of your lover's penis will bring you closer to orgasm; your man may find the squeezing muscles too irresistible to resist—succumbing to orgasm during the game!

Eventually, you can learn to control those muscles so adeptly that you and your man can share extended orgasms that seem to go on forever!

16

Aphrodisiacs, Love Elixirs, and Pleasure Enhancers

Power is the ultimate aphrodisiac.
—Former Secretary of State Henry Kissinger

When a woman taps into the sex goddess that lives within her, she is tapping into her power. You will find, as you become more and more of the seductress you want to be, that following the path you have chosen becomes more natural.

And in those moments—we all have them—where you need a little passion prompt, there are many holistic ways to increase your own horniness and help get your man into a state of love!

The term aphrodisiac is derived from Aphrodite, the Greek goddess of love and sex. Human beings have been looking for love and erotic power in a bottle for five thousand years, and there are about that many millennia worth of aphrodisiacs and love elixirs to show for it. Interestingly, the stuff that seemed to work on emperors and explorers of yore still work on men and women today. While some can be purchased in a bottle, others can be purchased in the produce or other sections in your supermarket.

Every seductress should know what her aphrodisiac options are. Modern women who believe in the power of the goddess find it useful to have knowledge of the kind of stimulants that can aid in their seduction strategy. You may never use them, and may never feel you have to, but the information is there!

Obviously, any concoction or aphrodisiac you try has to be done in the spirit of partnership, between consenting adults. I believe the seductress must participate in anything she has planned for a man so that her sexual energy vibration will rise to the same frequency as his—unless, of course, you are always highly sexed and your beloved needs a lot more encouragement! In some cases, where your man needs a passion boost in order to "rise" to the occasion, you may not need the altered or enhanced state that aphrodisiacs provide. But it is so much fun to try it!

Easy Love Potions for Him

If you are going to slip your man a mickey, make it a natural one that is sure to cause him no discomfort. Some sex-savvy women throughout history found results with some of the following tasty turn-ons for men.

- It is said that Henry VIII, known as one of the most virile men of his time, ate tons of *parsley*. English housewives who slipped the seemingly unsexy greens into hubby's food found that he became quite amorous. The famous lover Casanova loved women and he loved...*chocolate*. The sweet stuff has been known to stimulate the brain chemical phenyltethylamine (PEA), known as the "love hormone," and makes you feel so good that you feel like making love. A Hershey's Kiss is said to do wonders for raising the spirits, and certain body parts, because carbohydrates in sweets raise the brain's seratonin level and sweet foods generate a rush of endorphins.

❤ The Aztec warrior-king Montezuma was believed to be a virile lover. He never entertained his harem without a cup of *cocoa,* first. According to the "Cooking Couple," Ellen and Michael Albertson, authors of the *Cooking Couple,* and *He's a Fork, She's a Spoon,* during one Mexican ritual celebrating the chocolate harvest, two thousand cups of cocoa were served in gold goblets by naked virgins to the emperor and his court.

❤ According to legend, the Roman emperor Nero was treated to *goat's milk, cinnamon, and rosewater,* according to legend, which was shared with him by his wife, who believed in taking it internally and bathing in it.

Foods That Enhance Desire

The Cooking Couple say *caviar* is known to increase the libido. But here's a cheaper carnal treat: Studies have shown that *black licorice* can increase penile blood flow. You can buy a bag of licorice sticks or swirls for under two bucks in your local supermarket.

Phalliclike foods such as *bananas, cucumbers, asparagus, and carrots* can be fun foods to put you in the mood. *Oysters,* as well as any fish or food resembling the female genitalia, are believed to evoke a man's desire for the female. At the very least, such foods can create a stimulus response: Oyster equals vagina, and eating an oyster is like tasting the sweet petals of the female parts. It is totally possible that aphrodisiacs work on a psychological level just as much as, or more than, a physical level!

There are many common foods that are believed to stimulate sexual arousal and desire. *The Encyclopedia for Erotic Wisdom* lists cinnamon, garlic, wheat germ, honey, sesame, and goat's milk as erotic enhancers.

An uncommon food, and probably the last thing any woman wants to have to cook for a man, is...*brains.* Author Oscar Kiss-Maerth researched, and personally tested, the ancient belief that monkey brains significantly boost desire and virility.

While you're shopping for sex-stimulating goodies, make sure to cross the following *off* your list, as they are famous for their anaphrodisiac qualities, which means they might knock the wind right out of his sail. Arousal *nots* include: vinegar, lemonade, tobacco, and too much alcohol. You might also want to keep him out of the cold shower and avoid trying to mount him near any body of water, as cold H_2O has a tendency to shrink the possibilities for sexual play.

Medieval Customs for Seduction

According to *History Laid Bare,* women of the Middle Ages had a number of interesting aphrodisiacal practices that simply required the recycling of bodily fluids.

- Swallowing semen was considered a way in which a woman could make a man's love burn brighter for her. One sip and he was her love slave.
- Menstrual blood was used as an attention-getting aphrodisiac. Women would put their menstrual flow into their husband's food or drink, because it was believed to make men pay more attention to them.
- The custom of rolling food on their flesh and then feeding it to the beloved was also common. For example, it is said that some women order that dough be rolled and bread be prepared on their naked buttocks; once cooked, they'd feed it to their mates in hopes their sexuality would burn more.

Herbal Aphrodisiacs

Much of the information on aphrodisiacs and sexuality enhancing practices, in general, comes from Chinese, Arabic, Indian, and

Good Scents

Dr. Alan R. Hirsch of the Smell and Taste Treatment Research Foundation in Chicago, is a neurologist and psychiatrist who has conducted numerous well-received studies on the effect of scent on the brain. He details his findings and ways to incorporate them into your love life in his latest book, *Scentsational Sex: The Secret to Using Aroma for Arousal* (Element Books, 1998). He says his research on scents that turn men on pointed to two top aromas: Pumpkin Pie and Lavender. Applied on surgical masks to the noses of men in the study, Hirsch says those scents proved to increase penile blood flow by 40 percent. Other food scents that got blood flowing to all the right places included: cinnamon rolls, licorice, strawberry, vanilla, and donuts.

Although Hirsch doesn't market products with those scents, he says the aroma can be placed on a cotton ball and kept in a test tube. You just stick it under your man's nose and get him to sniff frequently!

When I tested out Dr. Hirsch's suggested scents, I dabbed them on my skin, under my beloved's nose, on the sheets, and on the lightbulb near the bed. Another method would be to have a picnic—leave the food near the bed to help arousal and then eat it together as part of your love play!

Greek sources, yet in modern life, more information on herbal aphrodisiacs is emerging from South America, home to many of the titillating herbs used to spice up one's love life.

Herbal aphrodisiacs are considered Cupid's natural answer to your passion prayers because they are legal, safe when taken properly, and often serve as dietary enhancers as well. You can purchase them in your local health food store.

How do they work? I asked my friend Dr. J. Terry Lesher to

explain. "Contained within the plants (from which the substances are extracted) are chemicals that either directly stimulate centers in our brain or indirectly stimulate them by causing the release of appropriate brain chemicals which either heighten arousal or mimic the chemicals released during arousal and also released during and after sex."

While most allopathic physicians will not touch the aphrodisiac question (such as, "Is it safe?"), you should run it by a health practitioner who is in the know before ingesting or imbibing. Lesher suggests gathering all the information you can on the aphrodisiac you'd like to try and then finding a reliable medical professional to discuss it with. He points out that just because something is grown in the ground doesn't necessarily mean all the things in it are good. Some herbal formulas may have naturally occurring toxic alkaloids in the plant matter.

Some of the products considered to be the most favored herbal sex enhancers on the market include:

- *ginseng* originating mostly in Korea, the type of ginseng differs for men and women because it increases stamina and virility
- *marapuama* cultivated in many Third World countries to improve erection and libido
- *avena sativa* mainly made of healthy green oats and proven to stimulate that loving feeling
- *ginkgo nuts* from the ginkgo balboa tree, the Japanese use it to make a tonic for men because of its anti-anxieties abilities
- *yohimbe* one of the most famous and popular herbs for men, it aids blood flow to the penis to help with erections
- *damiana* used to cure low sex drive and aid in menstrual problems
- *catauba* a famous Brazilian aphrodisiac plant known for stimulation of male sexual and urinary organs, as well as producing wildly erotic dreams

In addition to herbal aphrodisiacs, there are a number of elixirs and formulas that combine many of the above into a potent blend. These include:

- Love Life, a blend of Chinese herbs, which requires taking pills, as well as homeopathic drops, several times a day.
- Men's Essential Sex Tonic and Women's Essential Sex Tonic from Elixir Tonics & Teas in Los Angeles.
- Femme Vitale and Man Power come in tiny (and not too tasty) tonic bottles with tiny straws, from Golden Mountain Herbs in Badger, California.

Personal Testimony

To check out the possibilities for passion, my partner, Richard, and I took some aphrodisiacs for a test-drive.

We designated a "weekend of love" and selected yohimbe and damiana—respectively for "him and her"—because we felt these two herbs would best pave the way to our shared desire for lots of rolling around in bed, playful sensual contact, and intense sexual response and orgasms.

We had one week in which to imbibe our individual love potions before our three-day bedroom expedition to see how well the aphrodisiacs actually work. We're here to tell you…they actually work!

Since attraction, stamina, and desire were not issues for us, we went for sensation-enhancing herbs. We decided against ginseng, because its greatest strength is to perpetuate a more athletic and enduring sexual performance (not a problem). We had purchased avena sativa, but Richard remembered taking it for a month and having no result other than a horse's hankering for oats for breakfast (besides, we didn't need to be inspired to have a roll in the hay). We flirted with "Love Life," but the formula required more pill and drop popping then we had time for (it takes a while to kick in). Catauba, the herb we most lusted after, was the most elusive. We did everything short of fly to Brazil to try and locate it. We've heard through those who'd taken the world-famous Brazilian love herb that it causes wildly colorful, explicit erotic dreams—great for those nights when you have a warm body next to you in bed!

In general, a weekend in bed, and a good relationship and communication go a long way toward letting a good aphrodisiac enhance the experience. Yet, coming together after a week on love herbs made us ripe for new and exciting levels of pleasure and delight. Our lustful feelings seemed to have a robust power of their own, and the vigor of the Energizer Bunny. We kept on going and going and...

She Says

This was my introduction to herbal aphrodisiacs. Prior to this, I considered any man who let me talk for a half hour before sex to be the greatest aphrodisiac. Richard was all ears—and other willing body parts—and he supported and monitored my aphrodisiac intake. When doing aphrodisiac with a partner, it's important to communicate about who is taking what when, so that you can stay on the same arousal cycle.

The minute I slugged down my first eight drops of Damiana Leaf (Turnera aphrodisiac) I got that loving feeling, but I think my first response was mental. After a few days, however, I discovered that when I took Damiana I would lubricate luxuriously. Richard pointed out it was a good move to take some about twenty to thirty minutes before intended sexual activity. My female organs were so hypersensitive, I could feel the herb infiltrating my fallopian tubes, ovaries, and vulva. I was in a state of constant arousal. My partner's every stroke, every touch, permeated my body. I felt totally open and relaxed. My orgasms were amazingly easy and intense.

Most delicious was the mutual desire to be flesh against flesh with one another without needing time out. Richard was totally available and ready to engage at any moment. I really loved the way we were erotically magnetized to one another all weekend. We'd make love, take a break, make love, order food, make love, talk for a while, make love...

He Says

Richard sums up his experience as follows: "Attraction to your partner, as well as state of mind, impacts the experience. If you are already turned on to your partner, you can't always tell what feelings are stirred by this natural attraction and which sensations are aphrodisiac-induced. Used safely, I find that herbal love potions can enhance a good sexual partnership—as well as wake up a sleepy one—and give couples a fun erotic experiment they can partake in together.

"You've got to be willing to experiment to find the right formula, or mixture; some herbal aphrodisiacs work better in combination. It is specific to a person's body chemistry and the herb being used. From my experience with yohimbe, I know it's important to take it two or three times a day, to build up to the erotic experience; also, to take it forty-five minutes to a half hour before sexual activity. Taking it sublingually—liquid drops held under the tongue—is the most powerful method because it goes straight into the system.

"I noticed a shift in energy very quickly: Just thinking about making love moved a lot of feelings down to my groin. Once we were physically together, there was a qualitative difference in the timing of erections (quicker), as well as strength and endurance. An even greater drive, however, was my desire to simply touch, caress, and kiss her.

"Perhaps the most powerful aphrodisiac for me was Laurie Sue's response. In sex therapy, we call it the EPO (excitement, plateau, orgasm) and hers was amazing. Even the slightest touch—and I mean slight—generated an extremely passionate response. She was in a state of arousal, and didn't really require much from me to get there—my strongest role was being there for her. I think we both had extremely generous orgasms—there were many, each more intense and long-lasting—and lots of fun."

In general, Richard and I had a wonderful experience together. Clearly, good communication and shared intention go a long way. I think aphrodisiacs are for lovers—not for first-time dates. So if you include any of these love potions, elixirs, or herbal aphrodisiacs in your seduction repertoire, be respectful.

17

Becoming the Sacred Seductress

I think a man is always looking for a goddess.
—Deepak Chopra

The most important relationship you will ever have is the one you have with yourself. Sacred love is something that comes from within that you can share with another; it's not something that a man can create for you, or even with you. Until you love, respect, and treat yourself like a goddess—or as you would choose to be treated by a good man—that good man cannot get in your temple door.

That's why it is so important to develop, nurture, and bring out your true inner seductress. A silky shirt, red lipstick, and heels can easily seduce a man's eyes and body, yet when you are also expressing yourself from your heart and soul, you are laying the foundation for a conscious, loving relationship—with yourself and with your significant other. As you evolve, your partner will evolve or a more evolved partner will come your way.

Evolving as a Goddess

Your evolution as a seductress and sex goddess can move to the next phase if you choose: the phase of love goddess. This means elevating yourself to view yourself, your beloved, and your romance from a more expansive spiritual perspective. From that perspective, you are free and you are accepting; you are not manipulating your man out of fear that things won't go your way. You are fully engaged in your own life and your own development. And as you grow into the woman you want to become, you will allow your man to grow as well, and you will very naturally guide him to a point of loving connection where you can both truly engage in a relationship.

Like the revered sacred seductress—the sacred prostitute— you can open yourself to a man (the right man for you) and share with him your feminine power—and that will power your relationship. The archetype of the sacred seductress is that when she surrenders her ego and accepts a man without condition, he is magically transformed. In expressing our highest nature, we are meant to heal and nurture, teach and learn lessons in relationships. We are meant to leave open spaces in relationships in which people can grow and expand. Sexual expression is often the doorway to this kind of love.

"Of course, women can't flock to temples and set up camp as holy whores in this day and age without being arrested," points out Diana Rose Heartwoman in *Ecstasy Journal: The Journal of Divine Eroticism* (vol. 11, no. 3). "But a change in the way women view themselves and how men view women might be a start. Every woman can evoke the Holy Whore into her life with pleasure."

Heartwoman quotes Jungian psychologist Nancy Quall-

Corbette's description of the sacred seductress: "She is a woman who, through ritual or psychological development, has come to know the spiritual side of her sexuality, her true eroticism, and lives this out according to her personal circumstances. The Sacred Prostitute lives on all life's walks. She is a woman who has reclaimed herself and connected with her will. Most importantly, she is that woman who has reclaimed the sacredness of her body."

My favorite modern example of a sacred seductress is the role of Annie Savoy in the movie *Bull Durham*. Portrayed to perfection by actress Susan Sarandon, who has always publicly expressed her inner sex goddess, Annie honors the feminine, elevates sexuality to its highest form, and treats baseball as a religious experience. Utilizing her femininity, sexual openness, and metaphysics, she initiates one player per year to his own power—by sharing her female prowess. Her skillful seduction includes everything from cuffing a guy to the bed and reading poetry to him as a way of redirecting his sexual energy into his pitching, to actually holding baseball practice with these men. She chooses men—as opposed to them choosing her—whom she can believe in and validate. She serves the men of baseball as the sacred whores served men in the temples—and she is highly revered and respected for both her sensuality and her keen eye for the game.

Like all mortal women, Annie finds that beneath her seductive ability is a vulnerability. Eventually, she reveals this part of herself to the right man and evolves toward a more autonomous sacred relationship (with Kevin Costner!).

Confer With Your Love Goddess

Before you decide to move your relationship to the next level, meet your inner love goddess and see if she is ready to be as vulnerable and strong as a woman must be in order to be truly intimate with, and initiate, her man.

When you are authentic with yourself, you can then be real with another person. When you are committed to your own well-being, you can then be committed to the well-being of another. When you are truly intimate with yourself and know yourself beyond the masks of everyday living, then you can be intimate and engage with another. Often, when people evolve in those ways, they seek something more. They are seeking a soul connection.

As Deepak Chopra told me recently, "Unless you are in touch with the spirit you cannot maintain a loving relationship."

You can be playful, sexy, erotic, a turn-on—but if you want to truly share a sacred love, you have to be willing to bring yourself fully into a relationship. This is where the seductress becomes a true lover, a sex goddess becomes a love goddess; it is where seduction becomes sacred.

I am not talking about something that is out of reach, or too lofty and mythical to have meaning in our lives. It's part of our higher nature to tap into the gods and goddesses within. "I think that's the journey that we're undertaking," says Chopra. "Sacred, mysterious, and mythical characters are actually archetypes that represent states of our own being. So there's mythical ecstasy and then there's sacred ecstasy. When you have all three—physical, sensual/sexual, mythical/sacred—then you're in bliss."

Keeping Him Under Your Spell

The way to keep a man under your spell is to love his soul, as well as all he is as a man, and allow him to follow his own bliss. The way to allow a man his happiness is to make room for the little boy in him and let that little boy come out and play. It is the frustrated child who can't get what he needs who acts out, or withdraws, in relationships. What cuts men off from women is when we try to cut them off from themselves and the things they love.

What makes men stay—in a loving, fully present way—is

freedom. While it may sound contrary to "making a relationship work," it is not. A man needs to be accepted, validated, and supported by his woman—and gently guided elsewhere when he's off the track. He also has to be allowed to make his way in the world as a man. If he can trust you to leave his personality intact, and stop touching his posessions and trying to arrange them your way, he will quite naturally begin to grow in the direction you, as the great initiator, have set forth—but only if he's allowed to go at his own pace and walk on his own feet.

Give a man the space to do so and you may be amazed at what happens. Hold in your mind an image of him as you know he can be—without pushing him to become it—and you might find that with the help of your love he will become all he can be.

Think of the mother goddess, holding her child in the highest light, having faith in his vision and his quest. Mothers traditionally hold their boys in high esteem and offer wisdom that will shape them into quality men. The sacred seductress can also hold a man in the highest esteem as she continually seeks out his best qualities and acknowledges them, thus empowering him to create more of those qualities in himself.

Tantric Sex

The fastest way I know to find bliss, especially for women who have taken the path of the seductress, is to engage in the study and practice of the esoteric arts of love, for within these dwell the joy of the erotic and the connection of spirit. As it is said in the ancient text of the Kama Sutra, this is a place "where the ecstasy of lovers merging is the ecstasy of man touching God."

I started my search for bliss by exploring and unfolding my sexuality; then I continued my search for sex with soul. Ultimately, I found my way to a more intimate relationship with myself, and that opened the door to being with a man unlike any

I'd ever been with—a man who was capable of loving and who shared my hunger for the journey; a man who believed in sacred partnership before I even got there!

But evolution began with that gentle, gnawing feeling that there must be something more—that even though I've known orgasmic pleasure, it hadn't quite measured up to the rockets and rainbows, fireworks and shooting stars of romantic fairy tales. I knew in my gut that there was something more to lovemaking—but I had no way of comprehending what that possibly could be without reaching out to experience a sacred kind of love with a loving partner. I found that route through Tantric sex.

The basic premise of the ancient art of Tantric sexuality is this: couples who practice Tantra together share a deeper ability to communicate, a spiritual connection, and an extraordinary expression of erotic love. Although Tantra is devoted to honoring the female, both partners share in loving exploration of sexual pleasures. Tantric sexuality can unite intimate partners on all levels.

Most important for those not yet in the right relationship: It is possible to become educated and familiar with Tantric sex techniques—even if you don't have a partner—and practicing this spiritual approach to romantic love solo will prepare you for a relationship. When the appropriate partner comes along, you'll be ready. Success is when preparation meets opportunity. This applies in the laws of love and spirit as well.

Tantric sex for modern men and women has been brought into the twentieth century in "The Art of Conscious Loving" seminars taught by Charles and Caroline Muir, a Hawaii-based married couple who travel the country enlightening both couples and singles about practical ways to incorporate Tantric sexuality into their daily lives. "We've taken the original Tantric customs and have done our best to best to translate them to Judeo-Christian ethics," explained Charles Muir at recent seminar. "This course is designed to make you into a better kisser, lover, and toucher. It's also designed to make you a better communicator."

The Sanskrit word Tantra means "expansion," and relics of Tantric rituals date back nearly five millennia, although the Tantric texts (108 in total) didn't begin to appear until a few hundred years B.C., according to the Muirs.

Hindu practitioners of Tantric yoga practiced and taught sexual play and sexual union early on in life. "Tantra is a spiritual system," explains Charles Muir, "and in the Tantric teachings, sexual love is a sacrament. Tantra's goals, however, are broader in scope than simply to accomplish proficiency in sex. The ultimate goal is union with God, or the cosmic consciousness, or whatever you choose to call it. Focusing one's mind on one's partner and nurturing the relationship are at the heart of conscious loving. Therefore, the act of love is performed quite literally with premeditation. Conscious lovers designate a time in which they can comfortably engage in a love ritual without interference or stress."

Taking this conscious approach, as opposed to a "whatever happens happens" attitude, allows lovers to prepare themselves mentally, as well as logistically, by preparing a private, comfortable place for intimate exchange. This means the kids, the office, the stress of daily life will not be invading the boudoir.

Tantric practitioners of yore had unusual Hindu names for sex organs, which are still used today. The penis is called *lingam* and the vagina is *yoni*. Tantric lovers don't *penetrate*, rather they *enter*. Another key word is *permission*. The language is designed to treat the organs and acts of love respectfully.

The concept is that Tantra can elevate a couple's lovemaking to an art form and to a deep sense of spiritual connection. When this occurs, Tantric lovers feel totally connected to one another and to the source of life itself. It is a very loving and gentle practice that teaches eye and body contact, which serve to bring a couple into a closer state of intimacy and genuine togetherness.

Seek and Ye Shall Find... Your G Spot

The G spot has long been heralded as the elusive female love spot that truly can send you to new heights of passion. The ancient teachers of Tantric love and sex have been aware of this female pleasure spot for millennia, and it has been referred to as a sacred area. Charles Muir renamed it the "sacred spot."

The sacred spot—-which is literally the size of a pea—is located in the upper wall of the vagina. When stimulated, in conjunction with or separately from the clitoris, it arouses the female and she is capable of multiple orgasms and that mysterious, most coveted, controversial female ejaculation—in Sanskrit it is known as *amrita* or "divine nectar." The amrita doesn't emanate from the same place that most female fluids come from (such as the bartholin glands or the cervix); amrita is ejaculated through the urethra but it is not urine or mixed in with urine. It is female ejaculate.

For women, one of the first hurdles to jump is not just finding the G spot, but believing it actually exists! Up to 50 percent of gynecologists still insist there is no such thing as a G spot. In their seminar, the Muirs instruct participants on precisely how to locate it and stimulate it. Some women have difficulty accessing feeling in that part of their body. The process of bringing feeling into the area is called "sacred spot massage" and it enhances healing.

It is believed that the sacred spot functions in the genitals similarly to the way the subconscious mind functions in the brain—it is the keeper of all sexual records—your pleasure, your pain, your grief. Memories of old broken hearts, lost virginity, sexual abuse, and negative sexual experiences are stored in the spongy area that rests right behind the pubic bone.

Sharing the secrets of the G spot with a man while maintaining full eye contact is one of the most intimate experiences I have ever had. I can honestly say that working with the sacred spot has helped me heal. That is the truest possibility for sacred sexuality: to be healed of the pains of the past, the broken hearts of yesterday, the losses, and to be clear enough to access spirit. That's why they say it is like becoming one with God.

Sexual desire and response evolve with time, as you learn more about what you like, and your partner—if you have a steady one—figures out more ways to please you. Discovering Tantra, or any new practice, is about changing, growing, and being exposed to new things. It doesn't mean what you did before was bad—it's learning a new skill that will bring pleasure to both you and your sweetheart. To master G spot orgasms you have to give yourself time to learn and practice. A G spot orgasm has some of the same qualities as a clitoral orgasm—the building of excitement and the spreading of tingly feelings—yet it doesn't have the same sense of urgency. It grows above and beyond anything previously experienced and expected. Not only does the explosion of pleasure feel like it's shooting up toward your throat and moving sideways into the reproductive organs, it also is felt in the thighs and breasts. Most of all, it gives women a great sense of opening up and becoming more expansive.

Because Tantric sexuality is a woman-centered practice, many women feel safe, secure, and honored. The men attracted to Tantra are generally very conscious and spiritually inclined. They are also more emotionally available than most. As Caroline Muir points out, "This work involves them being very vulnerable and being willing to go into their emotions."

Because of the nature of Tantra, men and women find they are in an environment in which the normal male-female dynamics are not present. Everyone who engages in the learning process suspends their usual judgments and focuses instead on being in the moment.

"I felt so connected to everyone I did exercises with," said one woman who attended a Conscious Loving seminar. "I feel in love—well, a little bit in love—with a lot of men. But most of all, the way they treated me helped me fall in love with myself!"

Actors Jill Eikenberry and Michael Tucker, of *L.A. Law* fame, are among the couples who have found connection and bliss together through Tantric sexuality. In an interview with journalist Sara Davidson for *Mirabella* magazine, Eikenberry said that sacred spot work provided her with "an incredible release...a washing away of all kinds of things." She said the orgasmic pleasure of a sacred spot orgasm was far greater, and easier to achieve, than other kinds.

Tucker said, "It transformed the way we thought about sex. It took us to states we never imagined, and I realized: This is what we're here for, to love like this."

Tantra Tips for Lovers

There are elements to Tantra you can use anytime, such as eye contact. When you look deeply into someone's left eye, you connect with them intimately and immediately. This technique can help anyone develop immediate rapport in almost any situation. The Muirs also suggest the following tips:

- Take time for "ten-minute connects." At least once a day, couples should share a hug, touch, embrace, or a roll on the bed for ten short minutes. This will help enhance intimacy in relationships and keep couples connected.
- Take turns. Partners can switch roles regularly so that initiating sensuality in a relationship is a shared experience. This way, no one has all responsibility, and each partner has a chance to give, receive and experiment with what they want.
- Experiment. Learn what really feels good and pleases your partner by trying different sensual strokes, caresses, and

techniques.

- ♥ Kiss often. Use your lips to let your partner know how much you care. Alternate styles of softness, speed, pressure, and playfulness.
- ♥ Harmonize moods and energies. Lying down together quietly and breathing in unison is one way for couples to get on the same wavelength.

A Sacred Way to Keep Him Seduced

Men have a sacred spot too, and the woman willing to find it— and love it—gains the key to his heart. The male sacred spot is located inside the anus; it is similar to the woman's sacred spot in that it is a small, pea-sized area that, when stimulated, brings great pleasure. It may take some getting used to—especially for men who are not comfortable with anal penetration. Yet, like the female sacred spot, it can withstand more massage and stimulation than can a clitoris or penis.

But put away all your thoughts of what you think may happen and think of what you can make happen—you can pleasure your man beyond any measure, help heal him, and keep his prostate area healthy.

As Caroline Muir explains, a woman must relax her man with massage, soft music, and atmosphere. Make him feel safe and loved—and make sure he is willing to experiment. Using plenty of lubricant (such as Probe), she suggests the following:

Lay a man down on his back so that you can maintain eye contact. Have him raise his legs to give you access. Gently introduce your finger into his anus, gliding it in slowly. The sacred spot is right past the rim, in the vestibule right behind the opening. If he is on his back, and you kneel between him, you would hook your finger upward to reach the spot. Touch the spongy tissue and press and tap gently. This will begin to awaken his sacred spot. Do not confuse it with the prostate, which is a small, nut-sized organ located higher up. And do not expect an erection or an orgasm—although either could happen. This is not the time to focus on the penis.

If you can maintain eye contact with your man and massage that area, you will find him opening up to you more and more. He might become very emotional. If he does, let him express his feelings. If he is willing, he may have an emotional release. Encourage him to communicate and even cry. Gently—ever-so-gently—allow him his process. On the other side of his anger, fear, or sadness is the magnificent partner you have dreamed of. Beyond the places that need healing are places that are hot spots of ecstasy.

Many men initially feel uncomfortable with the idea of having something inserted in the anus, yet you will be surprised how they adapt to the feelings of joy and ecstasy that follow when a man allows his woman to offer such a healing. When eye contact is maintained, a couple shares a deeply intimate experience. A man learns to surrender to his woman and surrender to love.

He will fall in love with the goddess who can love him and share his ecstasy, and allow him to bring her the great joy of healing him and being healed by him. A woman who shares that kind of intimate contact with her man is a woman who can keep a man seduced!

Getting Closer to God (and Goddess)

In the Tantric arena, women are revered. Although offering a sacred-spot massage to your man is a wonderful gift of love, the ultimate gift you can give a man is your *amrita*—for what a man loves most is to please his woman. The amrita fluid is considered rich with the power of a woman because it contains the essence of the feminine—like perfume, this strong female nectar has an alluring quality.

It also has a healing quality: Charles Muir often tells men to put amrita on their face, like aftershave (when they receive such a gift from the goddess), for it contains a secret strength. Perhaps that is because a man who is permitted to come that close to his beloved knows in his heart that he has been accepted fully, that he is loved and appreciated, that he is trusted, that he has been let into her soul. When a woman shares it with her man, it is a sign that she is vulnerable enough to allow him to deeply touch her. Tantric masters very much consider love with a woman to be holy—it is a way for a man and a woman to get closer to God and goddess, and a way for them to be that for one another.

In Closing

You can't change the music of your soul.
—Katherine Hepburn

My work has led me to many adventures that have facilitated my growth and self-awareness. And I know that I chose my profession, and the sexuality specialty I followed for many years, as a way to access experience and insights that would contribute to my own transformation. I think I have always known, even before I *knew,* that a spirit who was guiding me every step of the way dwelled in me. Having been a student of seduction most of my life, I have in recent times added the role of teacher. Yet I am still a student—as we all are—because evolution requires an ongoing willingness to learn and grow. This ongoing openness is guided by the yearnings and desires of one's own spirit, even when it doesn't make total sense at the moment.

For example: When I first heard about Tantric sex I thought it sounded off the wall. Then it was intriguing…then it seemed to make sense…then I wanted to try it…then I couldn't imagine not knowing about it…then I could never consider a sexual experience that was not totally honorable and honest. What I am trying to say is that your seductress spirit will move you at the right pace if you let her, and your attitude will adjust in increments that you can accept.

If I could ask one thing of you it would be that you try not to be too critical of yourself as you travel the path of finding and expressing your inner seductress. It doesn't really matter where you come from. Focus on where you want to go. Getting there is the journey and the process. If you follow your heart and are true to yourself, you will find yourself on a gentler path. Remember: Seduction is supposed to be fun—not a struggle, not painful. Learn to distinguish the discomfort that sometimes comes with the experience of breaking through an inhibition you want to break through, and the discomfort that comes with following someone else's game plan.

I am one of those seductresses who evolved through stages of neediness, lust, and a soul-stirring need for self expression, finally reaching readiness for a connection to myself, and then with a man, that went way beyond the genitals. My intense curiosity led me to try many things, yet I am not all those things I studied as a seductress. Elements of things I know have blended with who I have become. I hope you are blessed with the same opportunities for development. The seductress in you is more than a sexpot; she is the spirit of your sensual, sexual self and she deserves to express herself fully in your life.

There's a wonderful saying that goes, "When the student is ready, the teacher appears." For many years, I believed seduction was just about sex. I had no clue of what was available with a man beyond the bedroom or what was possible in relationships when two people made themselves fully present and available to one another.

I was blessed with a wonderful physician who, at a point when I was questioning my sexuality, said: "Have you ever considered sex with love?" Until that moment, I hadn't. I thought they were two separate entities. I had developed my inner seductress, but not my spirit. It was at that moment that I took my first baby steps toward my inner sex goddess and began a journey that has led me deeper into the highest possibilities of love.

May you live your journey with great joy and wonder as you let your inner seductress out to play. Let her do what makes her heart sing. You deserve it!

APPENDIX

Safe, Responsible Seduction and Sex

It's no news flash that having multiple sex partners increases risk of sexually transmitted diseases (STDs)—simply because of possible exposure to bacterial and viral infections that the man carries or has been infected with by other sex partners. Even one partner can impact you based on his sexual style, habits, history, and honesty.

Familiarizing yourself with male anatomy, and knowing how STDs and other afflictions manifest in the male and can be transferred to the female, will put you ahead of the game. Don't be shy about talking sex with a guy (make it foreplay) and finding about his sexual history. Sometimes a man needs to feel desired and safe before 'fessing up, and you have to be willing to take the news—even if it's not great. During a very seductive dinner with a gorgeous guy she was crazy about, Lauren nearly keeled over when he said, "I have herpes and genital warts, and, as you can imagine, I hate having to tell women that...but that's where I'm at." When they decided to become intimate, he showed her the areas of his groin that could be affected if there was an outbreak and they practiced safer sex with the use of latex.

Whenever possible, get a good gander at his genital area before taking the plunge. Make it sexy...just undress him under good lighting, and as you caress and play with him, eyeball his penis, scrotum, and groin area. If you see anything that looks vaguely like an outbreak of something on his sexflesh—herpes, genital warts, something crawling—talk about it. He may not even know it's there and you could be doing him a favor by mentioning it. Put off sex play if there are any obvious or suspected maladies, and sort out your guidelines for safer sex. In general, make a mental map of his penis. Notice the veins, the little bumps, the way his sex skin looks, so in the future you'll be able to detect any changes.

It's also important to know how a man's body interacts with a woman's. Investigative health journalist and healer Gary Null, author of over fifty wellness books and host of a syndicated radio show, explains that the nature of sex can unfortunately heap a lot of bacteria on a woman. He suggests that couples always shower and wash with anti-bacterial soap before sex. For instance, even after washing with an antibacterial soap, fluids can leak from a woman's anus and be transferred to her vagina. "The number one cause of cystitis in America is a man's testicles hitting a woman's buttocks, and then the bacteria wiping across the woman's vagina and going into her urethra, and then into her bladder. Millions and millions of women each year get that."

Bone up on his body by reading *Men's Private Parts: An Owner's Manual,* by James H. Gilbaugh Jr., M.D. (Crown, 1993). Further educate yourself on safe-sex techniques by purchasing a book or, even better, a how-to video that spells out and shows the best way to have safer sex. *The Complete Guide to Safer Sex,* published by the Institute for the Advanced Study of Human Sexuality, comes in both book and video form. (See Resource Guide for ordering information.)

Of course, it goes without saying: Make sure you know your

own sexual health status before you embark on your journey to bring out the seductress within. Your conscious awareness of your own health—and health challenges—will help you to be a safe seductress.

Never hold back the truth about an existing STD from your lover—you have to be honest and up front from the start. You also have to be clever in order to make it more comfortable for both of you. Include revelations and confessions before either of you gets too hot to stop a sexual event in process (i.e., don't bring this up just as he's about to penetrate!) and present it along with the solution of how any conditions will be addressed during sexual play.

Finally, don't forget to practice birth control if it is your intention to enjoy sex without pregnancy. Some of the most adorable baby humans are born out of some of the wildly passionate nights you are about to engage in. Babies produced by this book will hopefully be planned-for and welcomed family additions, not by-products of irresponsible lust or casualties of unprotected sexual love.

You have not seen much lecturing about safe sex, STDs, and unwanted pregnancies in these pages. Take care of these essentials before you start so you can truly enjoy the delights of seduction!

Resource Guide

Following is a directory of books, videos, and audiotapes for seductresses.

BOOKS

Dating

The Complete Idiot's Guide to a Healthy Relationship, by Dr. Judy Kuriansky; Alpha Books (1998). A follow-up that shows the healthiest, happiest, hippest way to engage in a relationship.

The Complete Idiot's Guide to Dating, by Dr. Judy Kuriansky; Alpha Books (1997). Dr. Kuriansky's years of wisdom on dating and relating based on her work as host of the nationally syndicated *Love Phones* radio show.

Network Your Way to Endless Romance: Secrets to Meeting the Mate of Your Dreams, by Bob Burg and Laurie Sue Brockway; Samark Books (1997). Mail order only: 800-726-3667. A complete how-to on taking a businesslike approach to attaining a great romance. It includes an insightful clarification process called the Romantic Résumé that helps you declare what you seek in a mate.

Sexual Attraction and Attractants

Food as Foreplay: Recipes for Romance, Love, and Lust by the Cooking Couple; Alexandria Press (1996). A yummy collection of recipes and anecdotes about aphrodisiac food through the ages.

Intercourse: An Aphrodisiac Cookbook, by Martha Hopkins and Randal

Lockridge; Terrace Publishing (1997). Delicious edibles to set your heart on fire.

Love Cycles: The Science of Intimacy, by Winnifred B. Cutler, Ph.D.; Athena Institute Press (1991). A biological primer on pheremones, hormones, and how attraction comes about on the invisible chemical level.

Scentsational Sex; The Secret to Using Aroma for Arousal, by Alan R. Hirsch, M.D., F.A.C.P.; Element Books (1998). Evidence and tips on how certain scents can pep up your love life.

Searching for Courtship: The Smart Woman's Guide to Finding a Good Husband, by Winnifred B. Cutler, Ph.D.; Villard Books (1993). A practical, science-based explanation of how women can interact with men in a powerful, practical, and successful way.

Sex Appeal: The Art and Science of Sexual Attraction, by Kate and Douglas Botting; St. Martin's Press (1995). A compendium of information and examples of how attraction works.

Sex Tips

The Complete Guide to Safer Sex, by The Institute for the Advanced Study of Human Sexuality, comes in book and video. (Order from Open Enterprises, 800-289-8423.)

Every Woman's Guide to Sexual Fulfillment: An Illustrated Guide to Your Sexuality and Sensuality, by Susan Quilliam; Simon & Schuster (1997). This book briefly covers every topic relative to female sexuality.

The Good Vibrations Guide to Sex, by Cathy Winks and Anne Seamans; Cleis Press (1995). This is a bible of sex-positive insights that takes a healthy, clear, nonjudgmental approach to sex education about everything from sexual health to sex toys.

Sexsational Secrets: Exotic Advice Your Mother Never Gave You, by Susan Crain Bakos; St. Martin's Press (1996). A delightful exposé of the world of sensuality with tips, insights, and reporting on unique sensual opportunities.

Tricks: More Than 125 Ways to Make Good Sex Better, by Jay Wiesman (order from P.O. Box 1261, Berkeley, CA 94701). A popular list of sexual funsies, which is geared toward the S&M community but is insightful for anyone who wants to stretch a bit in their love life.

203 Ways to Drive a Man Wild in Bed, by Olivia St. Claire; Harmony

Books (1993). A best-selling compilation of tantalizing sex tips to try on your man.

Self-Esteem and Empowerment

Exhibitionism for the Shy, by Carol Queen; Cleis Press (1995). A how-to book of ways to unleash the exhibitionist in your soul.

Love 101: To Love Oneself Is the Beginning of a Lifelong Romance, by Peter McWilliams; Prelude Press (1995), 800-LIFE-101. Motivational and clear, this deeply stirring book looks beyond traditional self-improvement and into the realm of self-empowerment through personal responsibility.

30 Days to a Sexier You, by Paula Peisner Coxe and Jessica Daniels; Sourcebooks (1995). This is a cute, easy-to-follow book on a month's worth of self-esteem-enhancing exercises.

True Beauty: Positive Attitudes and Practical Tips From the World's Leading Plus-Size Model, by Emme with Daniel Paisner; G. P. Putnam & Sons (1996). An inspirational journey by a full-figured woman who made weight and size work for her. She shares her heartfelt belief that a woman who loves her body is a woman of power—no matter what her size.

The Goddess Within

Embracing the Goddess Within: A Creative Guide for Women, by Kris Waldherr; Beyond Words Publishing (1996). A who's who on goddesses that gives you a chance to see which ones you identify with.

The Goddess in the Bedroom: A Passionate Woman's Guide to Celebrating Sexuality Every Night of the Week, by Zsuzanna E. Budapest; HarperSanFrancisco (1995). A night-by-night, play-by-play manual of fun things to do with yourself and/or significant other.

The Goddess Oracle, by Amy Sophia Marashinsky and Hrana Janto; Element Books (1997). This combination book and deck of beautiful cards introduces you to fifty-two goddesses who can help you tap into the powerful feminine energy within and shows you how to change your life through easy-to-follow rituals.

Medicine Woman: A Practical History of Women Healers, by Elizabeth Brooke; Quest Books (1997). Capturing all aspects of feminine healing through history, this delightful manual shows how women have healed through the goddess, midwifery, love, and modern medicine.

Unleashing the Sex Goddess in Every Woman, by Olivia St. Claire; Harmony Books (1996). A book that declares there is a sex goddess within and that all women can be inspired by the goddess archetypes.

Sacred Sex

The Art of Conscious Loving, by Charles and Caroline Muir; Mercury House (1992). A classic on Tantric sexuality as interpreted and adapted for modern lovers by this world-famous teaching couple. Available through Source School of Tantra, 808-572-8364.

The Encyclopedia of Erotic Wisdom: A Reference Guide to the Symbolism, Techniques, Rituals, Sacred Texts, Psychology, Anatomy, and History of Sexuality, by Rufus C. Camphausen, Inner Traditions (1991). This amazing volume offers everything you need to know about erotic wisdom through the ages, with hundreds of fascinating descriptions and insights.

Sacred Sexuality, by A. T. Mann and Jane Lyle; Element Books (1995). An enlightening journey into the ancient esoteric teachings and history of sexuality.

Lasting Relationships

The Art of Living Consciously: The Power of Awareness to Transform Everyday Life, by Nathaniel Branden; Simon & Schuster (1997). This insightful guide to staying awake and aware in all you do gives clear and life-changing examples on where we "go unconscious" and how to stay present in our relationships.

The Couple's Comfort Book, by Jennifer Louden (Order from Isabella, 2780 Via Orange Way, Suite B, Spring Valley, CA 91978, 800-777-5205). A beautiful workbook of clarification and creation for couples who want to work things through together.

Journey of the Heart: Intimate Relationships and the Path of Love, by John Welwood, Ph.D., HarperPerennial (1990). Welwood's insights into relationships open a new door to conscious lovers who chose relationship as the path to evolution and growth.

The Path to Love: Renewing the Power of Spirit in Your Life, by Deepak Chopra; Harmony Publishers (1997). Chopra's key philosophy on loving supports the notion that we are beings with both dark and light sides, and yet we are most powerful when we maintain ourselves in a state of love.

Erotic Fiction

A Dangerous Day, by Charlotte Rose; Masquerade Books (1995). A meek and misunderstood housewife and new mom becomes a sexual dynamo and takes charge of her life in this erotic D&S themed novel.

The Doctor Is In, by Charlotte Rose; Masquerade Books (1994). A woman's journey from taboo to sexual wholeness through the eyes of a sensual female who makes love with all her doctors in order to learn how to heal herself.

Seductions, by Sincerity Jones; Masquerade Books (1991). A collection of eleven tales of lust from the female perspective designed to turn on women, seduce men, and provide tips for tantalization.

Women at Work, by Charlotte Rose; Masquerade Books (1992). Four sexy vignettes written in romance-book fashion that show how modern women make bold erotic choices. It was selected as one of the top five in women's erotic fiction by Dr. Ruth Westheimer in *New Woman* magazine.

Miscellaneous

The Couple's Guide to the Best Erotic Videos, by Steve and Elizabeth Brent; St. Martin's Press (1996). A husband and wife take a hands-on approach to reviewing sex films and write about their findings with recommendations for other married couples with kids.

His Secret Life: Male Sexual Fantasies, by Bob Berkowitz; Simon & Schuster (1997). The popular host of CNBC's *Real Personal* tells it like it is from the male point of view and invites women to understand what drives male sexuality and fantasy.

Men's Private Parts, by James H. Gilbaugh, Jr., M.D.; Crown (1993). An easy to read primer on penises, prostate glands, and more.

The Voyeur's Guide to Men/Women in the Movies, by Matt Martini; Contemporary Books (1994). A lively guide to sex, sensuality, and decadence in the movies.

VIDEO

Ancient Secrets of Sexual Ecstasy for Modern Lovers, Higher Love Video Series, P.O. Box 1818, Sebastapol, CA 95473, 800-9-TANTRA. Tantra brought alive through video demonstration.

The Bridal Shower, The Gift and other films by Candida Royalle; PHE

Distribution, 919-644-8100. Royalle is the country's premier director of erotic films from the female perspective, and her work always captures the essence of authentic female desire and pleasure while offering highly erotic sex scenes that couples love to watch together.

Cupid's Arrow: The Secrets of Love Potions, Aphrodisiacs & Spells, Central Productions. This video offers up a delightful and entertaining potpourri of erotic enticements that have served seductresses throughout history. Highly recommended.

Love Potions: A '90s Guide to Sexual Enhancement, with Cynthia Mervis Watson, M.D.; Xenon Entertainment. A video recipe book of aphrodisiacs.

Mary Magdalene: An Intimate Portrait, V.I.E.W. Video, 34 E. 23rd St., New York, NY 10010, 212-674-5550. This surprising documentary suggests that Mary Magdalene was unfairly dealt a historical "bad rep" and was in fact an extraordinarily powerful female force and ally to Christ.

The Secrets of Sacred Sex: A Guide to Intimacy and Loving, Living Arts, P.O. Box 2939, Venice, CA 90291-2939, 800-254-8464. Tantric sexuality and other esoteric sexual practices are explored and illustrated quite erotically in this how-to video. Fun to watch with a mate.

Sluts & Goddesses Video Workshop: Or How to Be a Sex Goddess in 101 Easy Steps, Higher Love Video Series, P.O. Box 1818, Sebastopol, CA 95473, 800-9-TANTRA. Former porn star and self-proclaimed New Age Girl Annie Sprinkle takes women on a journey of enlightenment to see how both the good and the whore within us all are beautiful creatures.

AUDIO

Sacred Fire: The Path to the Conscious Relationship, audiocassettes with John Welwood, Ph.D.; Sounds True, 735 Walnut St., Boulder, CO 80302, 800-333-9185. Get this audio to hear Welwood speak about his brilliant and transformational teachings on how relationships can be the foundation for extraordinary growth and development.

The Sex Goddess Within audio meditation with Laurie-Sue Brockway and sensual music by Doug Berlent; Media Right Music, 324 West 23rd Street, New York, NY 10011, 212-242-1039. Designed to help you evoke your inner sex goddess.

AUTHOR'S FAVORITE PRODUCTS

At-Home Tantra Training

This at-home training video shows soft, spirited, erotic communion, demonstrates how to develop an esoteric love match, and focuses on female pleasure that culminates in female ejaculation through "sacred spot" massage. *The Secret of Female Sexual Ecstasy,* produced by Charles and Caroline Muir, is a road map to woman-centered erotic loving. Set in Hawaii, it uses illuminating discussions and dazzling visual demonstrations to lay the groundwork for cultivating more spiritual relationships and engaging in lovemaking with gusto. Among the treats: sexual play in a Hawaiian waterfall; compelling scenes of how to massage a woman's sacred (G) spot; and hands-on training in female ejaculation in which Charles massages Caroline's sacred spot until she erupts in a waterfall amrita.

The underlying aim is to teach men how to approach relationships from this angle and show women how to be more receptive to being treated like a goddess. Order from Hawaiian Goddess, P.O. Box 69, Paia, HI 96779, 808-572-8364. Also available, the audio masterpiece, *Freeing the Female Orgasm,* with companion booklet.

Tantric Sex, to Go

Esoteric love and sex comes to you with these products. *The Tantric Massage Video* is fifty-eight minutes of sensual massage that makes you want to jump on the table and yell "Do me!" It shows graphic techniques for massaging the lips of the vagina, clitoris, nipples, penis, butt, et al. Also recommended, the *Secret Garden Trilogy,* which includes these books: *Tantric Massage,* a companion manual; *Sensual Ceremony,* which cues you on dozens of delicious feeding, bathing, bedroom, and sensual devotion rituals; and *Sacred Orgasm,* a beautiful book that focuses on the power of sexual energy, full-body orgasms, and sexual expression. Order from Pacific Spirit, 1334 Pacific Avenue, Forest Grove, OR 97116.

Tantra Wand

The Crystal Wand is a G spot stimulator that helps locate and massage the sacred spot area. Made of crystal-clear acrylic, it's ten inches long and is hand-carved into the shape of an S. It's shaped in such a way that it can easily reach the anterior wall of the vagina, where the G spot or sacred spot is found. With lubricant, it glides in easily and a woman can use it on her own, or with her mate. This area of the body is said to be the source of creative power for the female and the seat of Kundalini energy. Working the area with the Crystal Wand will help sensitize the body, release past wounds, and expand creativity, intimacy, and the connection to your mate. Order from Higher Love, P.O. Box 1818, Sebastopol, CA 95473, 800-9-TANTRA.

Erotic Training

Sexuality Seminars offers training around the country for people who want more from their relationships, and I highly recommend them. Instructor L. Lou Paget teaches a variety of sophisticated seminars that involve gathering around an elegant dinner table with beautiful china— and erotic toys. Women find rubber penises on their plates. Men find synthetic vaginas. In groups divided by sex, they learn extraordinary tips for pleasuring. You learn everything from amazing tongue tricks to how to properly lubricate a penis. Fun and safe, Paget does her seminars for bridal parties, corporate clients, and many, many Hollywood wives. For more information on having a seminar in your town, contact L. Lou Paget, 505 S. Beverly Dr., Ste. 198, Beverly Hills, CA 90212.

Index

Abuse, 16, 31, 89
Adam and Eve, 3, 4, 14, 74
Adult education courses, 67, 96
Albertson, Ellen and Michael
  Cooking Couple, 164
  He's a Fork, She's a Spoon, 164
Alcohol, 165
All in the Family (television series), 32
Amrita. See Female ejaculation
Ancient societies, 8–9
And God Created Women (film), 103
Antonelli, Laura, 96
Antony, Mark, 4–5
Anus, 148, 149, 182, 189
Aphrodisiacs, 30, 162–71
  favored, 133
  foods as, 164–65
  herbal, 165–68
  history of, 163–65
  personal testimony on, 168–71
  psychological aspects of, 164
  scents as, 5, 135, 139, 166
Aphrodite, 48, 162
Archetypes, 175
  goddess, 103, 113–14
  sacred seductress, 173
  slut, 113–14
  wild woman, 25
Art of Conscious Loving, The (seminars),
  Muir, Charles and Caroline 177–84
Attitude, 63–68
  of dominatrixes, 87, 90

of femmes fatales, 72–73
importance of, 65
See also Communication
Aural sex, 136–38
Avena sativa, 167, 168
Awakening ritual, 133–34

B&D (bondage and discipline), 7–8, 85
"Baby, You're a Star" (song), 121
Bacteria, 189
Baker, Josephine, 10
Bakos, Susan Crain, *Sexational Secrets:*
  Exotic Advice Your Mother Never
  Told You, 148
Barbarella, 4, 30, 66, 68, 102
Barbarella (film), 28, 66
Bardot, Brigitte, 103
Barrow, Sidney Biddles, 52
Basic Instinct (film), 49, 74
Basinger, Kim, 28, 84
Beatty, Warren, 6
Beauty ritual exercise, 36
Belly dancers, 79–80
  See also Strippers
Bening, Annette, 6, 74
Berkley, Elizabeth, 84
Berlent, Douglas, 137
Beverages
  Cleopatra's Elixir of Everlasting Love,
  134–35
  sensual brews, 135
Bible, 4, 11

Birth control, 190
Biziou, Barbara, *Joy of Ritual, The,*
    132–36
Blackman, Honor, 98
Blackwell, Elizabeth, 13
Black Widow (film), 74
Black widow spider, 70
Blame It on Rio (film), 104
Blaze (film), 84
Bleeth, Yasmine, 99
Blond bombshells, 100, 103
    See also Sexpots
Body & Soul Productions, 152
Body of Evidence (film), 71
Body Heat (film), 49, 71, 74
Bolton, Michael, 121
Bonaparte, Napoleon, 5
Bondage and discipline (B&D), 7–8
Bond, James, 98
Bottoms and tops, 95
Brain chemicals, 167
Braxton, Toni, 99
Breasts and cleavages, 56
Breathing in awakening ritual, 133
Brooke, Elisabeth, "Goddess as Healer,"
    8
Bugsy (film), 6
Bull Durham (film), 26, 28, 49, 174
Bullock, Sandra, 28
Burton, Richard, 32

Camphausen, Rufus C., *Encyclopedia of*
    Erotic Wisdom, 9, 70, 164
Candles, 140–41
Carey, Mariah, 99
Casanova, 11
Catauba, 167, 169
Cat Woman, 26, 101
CD-ROM, *Ultimate Sex Guide* (Hooper),
    154–55
Celebrities, 66
Celibacy, 14
Central Productions, 134–35
Cervix, 179
Channing, Stockard, 101
Childbirth, 158
Childhood, 31, 108

Chippendales (male strippers), 28
Chopra, Deepak, 21, 172, 175
Cinnamon roll scent, 166
Circle-jerks, 156
Cleavages and breasts, 56
Cleopatra, 4–5, 26, 69
Cleopatra and Caesar, 4, 7, 17
Cleopatra (film), 74
"Cleopatra's Clutch". *See* Pubococcygeus
    (PC) muscle
Cleopatra's Elixir of Everlasting Love
    (beverages), 134–35
Clitoris
    "clit," 127
    and the G spot, 156, 179, 180
    sex words for, 129–30
    vibrator stimulation of, 148–49, 150
Close, Glenn, 99
Clothing. *See* Wardrobe
Coaching on temptress traits, 67
Coccyx, 157
Cock, 124
Codependence, 73, 88, 89
Cohn, Richard A., 15, 159
Collages, 48–49
Collective unconscious, 12, 20, 55
Colors, 141
Comfort zone
    expanding, 39, 46–47
    for hot talk, 127
    and practicing, 67–68, 74
    and shyness, 109, 113
    starting in, 22–23
    of strippers, 82, 83
Communication
    sensual expression as, 12
    and Tantric sex, 178
    See also Attitude; Hot talk
Complete Guide to Safer Sex, The (video
    and book), 189
Computer therapy session, 155
Conception, 16
Condoms, 120
Conservative forces, 10, 14
Control and dominatrixes, 94
Cooking Couple (Albertsons), 164
Cosmic consciousness, 178

Costello, Lou, 85
Costner, Kevin, 26
Crawford, Joan, 70
Creating the environment, 120, 132–42
    aural sex, 136–38
    candles, 140–41
    colors, 141
    Feng Shui, 138–42
    flowers, 141
    lighting, 139–40
    ritual of awakening, 133–36
    scent, 139
    soft, sensual touch, 142
Crimes of Passion (film), 96
Crystals, 140
Cultures
    and Madonna/whore complex, 20–22
    sexual expression in, 14
*Cupid's Arrow: The Secrets of Love
    Potions, Aphrodisiacs and Spells,*
    134–35
Curtis, Jamie Lee, 64
Cystitis, 189

D&S (dominance and submission), 7–8,
    85, 87
Dafoe, Willem, 71
Damiana, 167, 168, 169
Damn Yankees, 52
Damsel in distress, 98, 102
    See also Sexpots
"Dance of Enticement" (Indian culture),
    79
Dance. *See* Exotic dance and dancers;
    Strippers
Dark and light sides, 20–22
"Dating Coach of the 1990s, The"
    (Moore), 68
Davidovich, Lolita, 84
Davidson, Sara, 181
Davis, Bette, 70
Deity, 8–10
    female, 70
Delany, Dana, 96
Designing Your Happiness (Wydra), 138
Desires, discovering, 38–50
Dickinson, Angie, 74

Dictionary of sex words, 127–30
Dildoes, 144
Dirty talk. *See* Hot talk
Diversity, sexual, 14
Divine Mother, 8
"Do Me Baby" (song), 121
Dominance and submission (D&S), 7–8,
    85
Dominas, 85, 93
    See also Dominatrixes
Dominatrixes, 26, 85–96
    and lifestyle, 85, 88, 93
    methods of, 86, 92
    temptress traits of, 94–95
    training course for, 91, 93–94
Domination parlors, 67, 87
Donut scent, 166
Double standard, 11
Douglas, Michael, 99
Dressed to Kill (film), 74
Dressing up and going out, 68
Dungeon, 86, 90–91, 93
    See also Dominatrixes
Dynasty (television series), 32

Early life experiences, 31
Ecstasy (CD), 137
*Ecstasy: The Journal of Divine
    Eroticism,* 9, 173–74
Eggs and sperm, 16
Eikenberry, Jill, 181
Ejaculation. *See* Female ejaculation;
    Semen
Element Books, 166
Elixir Tonics & Teas, 168
Encyclopedia of Erotic Wisdom
    (Camphausen), 9, 70, 164
Endorphins, 164
Enhancing Sensual Pleasure (CD),
    "Subliminal Soundtrack for
    Consenting Adults," 137–38
Environment. *See* Creating the
    environment
EPO response, 170–71
Erection, "hard-on," 127
Erotica (audiotape), 136
Erotic language. *See* Hot talk

Erotic writing, 39–47
Escort services, 52
Essex Entertainment, 136–37
Estefan, Gloria, 121
Etruscans, 79
Eulenspeigel Society, 96
Euphemisms for sexual organs, 127
Evans, Dixie, 79
Eve's Garden (sex boutique), 144
Excitement, plateau, orgasm (EPO) response, 170–71
Exhibitionism for the Shy (Queen), 108–9
Exhibitionists, 108–14
Exit to Eden (film), 88, 96
Exotic dance and dancers, 5, 14, 76–77
seduction of, 79–81
tempress traits of, 81–83
See also Eye contact; Private dance; Strippers
Eye contact
in erotic dancing, 77–82, 84, 116, 117, 120, 122
in G spot massage, 179–80, 183
in Tantric sex, 181

Fallen woman, 3
Fantasies
discovering, 38–50
in exotic dancing, 78, 80, 81, 83
and hot talk, 126
in *Hypnosex* program, 155
living out, 23, 27
men versus women, 17
ritual of awakening, 133–36
secret, 29, 39
writing about, 39–47
Fantasy engineers, 85
See also Dominatrixes
Fast women, 100–101
See also Sexpots
Fatale, Fanny, 156
Fathers, 31
Fears
and attitude, 66
of female sexual demons, 70
of losing control, 19–20

of Madonna/whore complex, 20–22
Female ejaculation (*amrita*), 109–10, 179, 183–84
Female inhibition, 6
Female praying mantis, 70
Femme Productions, 19
Femmes fatales, 11, 26, 69–75
definition of, 69–70
ice queen, 5, 71–72
temptress traits of, 72–74
Femme Vitale (aphrodisiac), 168
Feng Shui: Book of Cures (Wydra), 138
Feng Shui, 138–42
Feng Shui for Singles (Wydra), 138
"Fever" (song), 121
Field trips for observing temptress traits, 67, 96
Fifties, the, 7
Films
dominatrixes in, 95–96
femmes fatales in, 74
learning from, 49, 66
for self-love, 146
striptease in, 84
X-rated, 14
See also Videotapes
Fiorentino, Linda, 71–72
"Fire 'n' Desire" (song), 121
Fisher, Carrie, 104
Fleming, Rhonda, 84
Fleshlight (sex toy), 153–54
Flex-a-Pleaser, 150–51
Flowers, 141
Fonda, Jane, 4, 28, 30, 66
Foods that enhance desire, 164–65
Foreplay, 83, 137, 188
Foster, Jodie, 104
Frederick's of Hollywood, 82, 101
French tickler, 148
Function of the Orgasm, The (Reich), 13–14

Gadinia, 133
Game of seduction, 60, 86
Games Partnerships Ltd., Inc., 154
Garbo, Greta, 5, 74
Garden of Eden, 3, 74

Gaye, Marvin, 121
Genital warts, 188
"Georgia" (song), 121
Gift, The (video), 146
Gilbaugh, James H. Jr., *Men's Private Parts: An Owner's Manual,* 189
Gilda (film), 28, 104
Ginko nuts, 167
Ginseng, 167, 168
Goddess, 103
and God, 8–10
See also Sacred seductress
"Goddess as Healer" (Brooke), 8
Golden Mountain Herbs, 168
Goldfinger (film), 98
Gone With the Wind (film), 28, 32
Good Vibrations (sex boutique), 144, 149, 160
Gray, John, *Men Are From Mars, Women Are From Venus,* 52
Grease (film), 101
Griffith, Melanie, 104
Grifters, The (film), 74
Groin area, 189
Grold, Kevin, *Hypnosex* (audiotape), 155–56
G spot, 59, 145, 149
location of, 156, 179–81
and male PC muscle, 160
Gypsy (film), 84

Halloween, 110
Halpern, Steven, 137–38
Hanny Caulder (film), 69
Harris, Frank, *Love in Athens,* 136
Hayworth, Rita, 28, 104
Health food stores, 134, 166
Heartwoman, Diana Rose, "Musing on the Sacred Whore," 9, 173–74
Hellfire (S&M club), 96
Henry VIII, 163
Hepburn, Katherine, 32, 185
Herpes, 188
He's a Fork, She's a Spoon (Albertsons), 164
Hill, Virginia, 5–6
Hindu names for sex organs, 178

Hirsch, Dr. Alan R., *Scentsational Sex: The Secret to Using Aroma for Arousal,* 166
History Laid Bare, 165
Home Improvement (television series), 12, 32
Home stripping. *See* Private dance, at home
Honeymooners (television series), 32
Hooper, Ann, *Ultimate Sex Guide* (CD-ROM), 154–55
Hot talk, 123–31
erotic vocabulary, 128–30
female and male genitalia, 125–26, 128, 129–30
Houghton Mifflin, 155
How to Female Ejaculate (video), 109–10, 156
"How to Strip for Your Man" (stripping course), 117–18
Hurt, William, 49, 71
Hymen, 33
Hypnosex (audiotape), 155–56

Ice queen, 5, 71–72
See also Femmes fatales
"I'm So Excited" (song), 121
Incontinence, 158
Indiana, Mistress Tara, 86, 87, 91, 93–94, 111
Indian culture, 79
Inhibition, female, 6, 39
Inner seductress
beauty ritual, 36
embracing the dark and light, 20–22
evolutionary process in becoming, 22–23
finding your, 19–37
personal history review, 31–34
personal seduction scale, 27–30
power of a woman, 26–27
seductress summary exercise, 34–37
tips on bringing out, 47–50
wild woman within, 20, 24–25
See also Sacred seductress; Seductress
Institute for the Advanced Study of Human Sexuality, 189

Interactive Life Forms, 154
Intercourse. *See* Sexual intercourse
Internet sex, 59
Intimacy (CD), 137

James, Rick, 121
Jasmine, 133, 135
Jesus Christ, 11
Johnson, Michelle, 104
Jong, Erica, 10
Josephine, 5
Joy of Ritual, The (Biziou), 132–36
Judeo-Christian ethics, 177–78
Julius Caesar, 4

Kama Sutra, 176
Kama Sutra (film), 84
Kegelcisors, 159–60
Kegel, Dr. Arnold, 158
Kegel exercises, 158–61
Kinky sex, 39
Kissinger, Henry, 162
Kiss-Maerth, Oscar, 165
Kitten With a Whip (film), 102
Kuriansky, Dr. Judy, 111

L.A. Law (television series), 181
Lamarr, Hedy, 74
Lane, Lois and Superman, 98
Language. *See* Communication; Hot talk
Lap dance, 77
    See also Strippers
Last Seduction, The (film), 71–72
Las Vegas, 6
Latex, 188
Lavendar scent, 166
Lawrence, D. H., 97, 136
Leave It to Beaver (television series), 32
Lee, Gypsy Rose, 79, 107
Lee, Jennie, 79
Lee, Pamela Anderson, 99
Lee, Spike, 13
Leigh, Vivien, 28
Lenny (film), 84
Lesher, Dr. J. Terry, 166–67
Lessons on temptress traits, 67
Liberated women, 10, 20
Licorice scent, 166

Life Publications, 156
Lighting, 139–40
"Like a Virgin" (song), 108
Linton, J. P., 136
Little Egypt, 84
"Little Red Rooster" (song), 121
Living spaces, 138–42
Lolita (film), 104
Lolitas, 102, 104
    See also Sexpots
Long, G. G., 119–21
Love in Athens (Harris), 136
Love elixirs and potions. *See*
    Aphrodisiacs
Love hormone, 163
Love Life (aphrodisiac), 168
Love muscle. *See* Pubococcygeus (PC)
    muscle
Lovers Swing (sex toy), 152
Love and sex, 18, 186–87
Love Story Classics, 136
"Love Toy" (song), 121
Loy, Myrna, 95
Lubricants, 182
Lusty Lady (strip club), 79
Lyon, Sue, 104

McDowall, Andie, 28, 98
McPherson, Elle, 99
Madonna, 6, 11, 22, 28, 70, 71, 98, 100,
    107, 121
Madonna/whore complex, 20–22
Magdalene, Mary, 11, 69
Magic Christian, The (film), 96
Males. *See* Men
Man Power (aphrodisiac), 168
Mansfield, Jayne, 6, 84, 98, 100, 103
Mantra, visual, 35–37, 48
Marapuama, 167
Mardi Gras, 110
Margret, Anne, 102
Marital aid, 143
    See also Masturbation
Mary Magdalene: An Intimate Portrait
    (video documentary), 11
Mary Magdalene, 11, 69
Mask of Fu Man Chu, The (film), 95

Masquerade Books, 127, 128
Masturbation, 15, 42
  with vibrators, 143–44
  on video, 109–10
  See also Self-love
Mata Hari, 5, 69
Mata Hari (film), 5, 74
Mating, women and, 12, 13
Media messages, 24, 48
Media Right Music, 137
Medicine Woman, 8
Medieval customs for seduction, 165
Men
  and aging, 102
  choices of, 51
  connections to, 13
  conversations with, 58–59
  domination by, 6–7, 13
  domination of, 85–96
  easiness of seducing, 52, 53, 65
  emotional release of, 183
  fantasies of, 17, 59
  in game of seduction, 60, 86
  genetic programming of, 12, 55
  getting attention of, 24, 27
  initiation to sex by women, 15–17
  keeping them seduced, 175–76,
    182–83
  kegel exercises for, 160–61
  matching fantasies with, 46, 64
  and the modern seductress, 51–60
  and monogamy, 14
  nature of, 3, 55–60
  sacred spot in, 148, 182–83
  sexual histories of, 188
  sexual manipulation of, 7–8
  transformation of, 173
  wrong ones, 49–50, 53–55
*Men Are From Mars, Women Are From
  Venus* (Gray), 52
Men's Essential Sex Tonic (aphrodisiac),
  168
Men's Private Parts: An Owner's Manual
  (Gilbaugh), 189
Menstrual blood, 165
Middle Ages, 165
Middle-Eastern culture, 79

Mirabella (magazine), 181
Mistresses, 85
  See also Dominatrixes
Monogamy, 14
Monroe, Marilyn, 6, 10, 28, 98, 100, 103
Montezuma, 164
Moore, Demi, 84, 119
Mostel, Zero, 115
Mozart, Wolfgang Amadeus, 136
Muir, Charles and Caroline, *The Art of
  Conscious Loving* (seminars)
    177–84
Music, 103
  in mood setting, 136–37
  for stripping, 120, 121
Music for Lovemaking, 137
Music for Lovemaking II, 137
Musing on the Sacred Whore
    (Heartwoman), 9, 173–74
Mythology, 103

Nakedness, 56, 57
Napoleon Bonaparte, 5
Nasstoys, 149
Natural sensuality versus physical
    beauty, 24
Neptune's daughters, 98
Nero, 164
Newsweek, "Science Wars, The," 16
New York magazine, 87
Nin, Anaïs, 10
9½ Weeks (film), 28, 94
Nipples, 149, 150
Norris, Chuck, 89
Null, Gary, 189

Obsessions, 38–39
Odyssey, 98–99, 103
Olisboi, 144
"Once" (Lawrence), 136
Orgasms
  descriptions of in hot talk, 125
  female, 16, 146
  and the G spot, 156, 179, 180
  male, 158
  and PC muscle, 161
Original sin, 4

Orloff, Judith, *Second Sight*, 25
Oshun, Yoruba River Goddess, 48

Passion (CD), 136–37
PC muscle. *See* Pubococcygeus (PC) muscle
Penis
  examination of, 189
  lingam, 178
  and pubococcygeus (PC) muscle, 157–58
  sex words for, 129
People with disabilities, 154
Perfect (film), 64
Performance anxiety, 111, 114
  in stripping, 118
Perrine, Valerie, 84
Personal history review, 81–34
Personal massager, 143
  See also Masturbation
Personal seduction scale, 27–30
Phallic-like foods, 164
Phenyltethylamine (PEA), 163
Pheromones, 5, 25
Phone sex, 59
Physical beauty versus natural sensuality, 24
Pieces Pearl (sex toy), 149–50
Playgirl, 53, 92, 127, 128, 146
Pleasure enhancers. *See* Aphrodisiacs
Pocahontas and John Smith, 4
Pointer Sisters, 121
Polygamists, 14
Pornographer's Dictionary, 128–30
Power of women. *See* Women, power of
Pregnancy, 16, 190
President of the United States, 52, 54
Presley, Elvis, 102
Pretty Baby (film), 104
Pretty Poison (film), 74
Priestesses, 9
Primal urges, 12
Prince, 121
Private dance, 77, 80, 83–84
  at home, 115–22
  See also Strippers
Professional sex workers, 13, 15, 24, 58, 64

Prostate gland, 145, 182–83
Prostitution
  sacred, religious, ritual, or temple, 9
  See also Professional sex workers
Pubococcygeus (PC) muscle, 155–56, 157–61
Pumpkin pie scent, 166
Pussy, 124
"Pussy Galore," 98

Quall-Corbette, Nancy, 173–74
Queen, Carol, *Exhibitionism for the Shy*, 108–9, 110, 112–14

Rabbit, Jessica, 103
Rabbit Pearl (sex toy), 150
Rankin, Wayne, 76
Rape, 16
Rapture (CD), 137
Reich, Wilhelm, *The Function of the Orgasm*, 13–14
Relationships
  sacred, 9, 18, 21, 174–84
  traditonal male-female, 8, 180
  with wrong men, 49–50, 53–55
Religious prostitution, 9
Richards, Patricia, 12
Rite of passage, 9
Ritual of awakening, 133–34
Ritual prostitution, 9
Robbins, Tim, 49
Role models, 11
  for dominatrixes, 95–96
  favorite, 28
  for male behavior, 31
  for seductress qualities, 65–66
  Titans of Temptation as, 68
Rolling Stones, 121
Roman culture, 14, 79
Romantic Sensations (sex game), 154
Roses, 141
Rourke, Mickey, 84
Royalle, Candida, 19, 41–42, 146
Russell, Theresa, 70, 74

S&M clubs, 63, 96
S&M (sadomasochism), 7–8, 85, 87

Sacred Prostitute, 9, 11, 173, 174
Sacred relationships. *See* Relationships
Sacred seductress, 8–10, 172–84
  evolving as a Goddess, 173–75, 185
  Tantric sex, 176–84, 185
  See also Inner seductress; Seductress;
Spirituality
Sacred spot. *See* G spot
Sadomasochism (S&M), 7–8, 85, 87
Safe sex, 59, 188–90
Salt 'n' Pepa, 121
Samson and Delilah, 4, 17
Samson and Delilah (film), 74
Sarandon, Susan, 26, 28, 49, 174
Saturday Night Fever (film), 140
*Scentsational Sex: The Secret to Using
  Aroma for Arousal* (Hirsch) 166
Scent. *See* Aphrodisiacs
"Science Wars, The," *Newsweek*, 16
Scores (strip club), 15
Scrotum, 189
Second Sight (Orloff), 25
"Secret Garden" (song), 121
Seduction
  of dance, 79–81
  easiness of, 52, 53, 65
  and love, 18, 186–87
  sacred, 8–10
Seduction (CD), 136
Seduction manual, 64
Seduction scale, 27–30
Seduction shyness, 107–14
Seduction signature, 63–68
  discovering, 60
  and hot talk, 124
  personal dance in, 79
Seductress
  checklist of qualities, 44–45
  definition of, 11
  knowing yourself as, 19–37
  and modern men, 51–60
  sex rules for, 55–60
  shrine to, 48
  tips on bringing out, 47–50
  unleashing of, 38–50
  See also Inner seductress; Sacred
    seductress

Seductress summary exercise, 35–37
Self-awareness, 26, 51, 54
Self-esteem, 109
Self-hypnosis, 155–56
Self-love
  ritual of awakening, 133–36
  sex toys for, 146–47, 149–51
  See also Masturbation
Semen, swallowing, 165
Sense of touch, 142
Sensual Lovers Ring (sex toy), 151–56
Seratonin, 164
Seven-Year Itch, The (film), 103
Sex in America: The Definitive Study, 14
*Sexational Secrets: Exotic Advice Your
  Mother Never Told You* (Bakos) 148
Sex clubs, 67, 87, 96
*Sex Facts: The Handbook for the
  Carnally Curious*, 144
Sex goddess. *See* Goddess; Seductress
Sex industry, 14
Sex kittens, 102, 104
  See also Sexpots
Sexpots, 97–104
  temptress traits, 103–4
  varieties of, 98
Sex rules for seductresses, 55–60
Sex scandals, 52
Sex shops, 96
Sextette (film), 103
Sex toys, 95, 143–56
  benefits of, 145
  for couples, 151–56
  for self-pleasure, 146–47, 149–51
Sexual arousal
  and hot talk, 124
  and pubococcygeus (PC) muscle, 159
  sex words for, 130
  See also Aphrodisiacs
Sexual diversity, 14
Sexual expression
  as communication, 12
  in cultures, 14
  and love, 186–87
  as a sacrament, 178
  of strippers, 82–83
"Sexual Healing" (song), 121

Sexual intercourse, 9
and dominatrixes, 86
initiation of men by women, 15–17
music for, 137
and PC muscle, 160–61
sex words for, 130
Sexuality, Intimacy, and Relationship
Enrichment Network (S.I.R.E.N.),
15
Sexually transmitted diseases (STDs),
188–90
Sexual manipulation as survival
mechanism, 7
Sexual revolution, 9–10
"Sexy Noises" (song), 121
Shampoo (film), 104
She's Gotta Have It! (film), 13
Shields, Brooke, 104
Showgirls (film), 84
ShowTime Waterproof Brush Massager
(sex toy), 153
Shubin, Steve, 154
Shyness. *See* Seduction shyness
Siegel, Bugsy, 6
Silverman, Jonathan, 100
Sirens, 98–99, 103
See also Sexpots
"Sluts and Goddesses" (workshop),
113–14
Slutty girls, 100–101, 103–4
See also Sexpots
Smell and Taste Treatment Research
Foundation, 166
Social institutions, 13–14
Something Wild, 104
Soul connection, 78, 175
See also Sacred seductress
Sperm and eggs, 16
Spirituality, 21
See also Sacred seductress
Sprinkle, Annie, 113
Stamford Hygienic, 149, 156, 160
Stanwyck, Barbara, 70
Stealing Home (film), 100
Stone, Sharon, 28, 49, 70, 74, 94
Strawberry scent, 166
Streetcar Named Desire, A (film), 32

Strip clubs, 63, 67, 76, 83, 115, 119
Strip courses, 117–19
Strippers, 76–84
burlesque-style, 79
tempress traits of, 81–83
See also Exotic dance and dancers;
Eye contact; Private dance
Striptease, art of, 82, 115
Striptease (film), 84, 119
Subconscious mind, 12, 22, 35, 138, 155
Subliminal media messages, 24, 48
"Subliminal Soundtrack for Consenting
Adults," *Enhancing Sensual
Pleasure* (CD), 137–38
Sultans and harems, 14
Superman and Lois Lane, 98

Table dance, 77, 80, 83–84
See also Strippers
Taboo, 14
sex toys as, 144
slutty women as, 100
Tantric sex, 43, 148, 176–84, 185
history of, 178
tips for lovers, 181–82
workshops and seminars, 63, 177–84
Taste sensations, 135–36
Taxi Driver (film), 104
Taylor, Elizabeth, 32, 74
Tchaikovsky, Peter Ilyich, 136–37
Teasing by dominatrixes, 86–87, 92, 95
Temptress traits
of femmes fatales, 72–74
tips for adapting, 66–68
Testicles, 149, 189
Thorn Birds, The (film), 104
Titans of temptation
as role models, 68
See also Dominatrixes; Femmes fatale;
Sexpots; Strippers
Tobacco, 165
Too Hot to Handle (film), 84
Topping from below, 7–8
Tops and bottoms, 7–8, 95
Toys. *See* Sex toys
Tracey, Spencer, 32
Transformation, 21, 35, 185

and self-awareness, 26
Travolta, John, 64
Tucker, Michael, 181
Turner, Kathleen, 49, 71, 74, 75, 96

Urethra, 189
Urine flow control, 157
Uterus, contractions of, 16

Vagina, 189
    fear of being lost in, 70
    and pubococcygeus (PC) muscle,
        158–61
    in ritual of awakening, 133
    sex words for, 129–30
Vamps, 101–2, 104
    See also Sexpots
Vanilla scent, 166
Varma, Indira, 84
Vault (S&M club), 68, 92, 96
Venus in Furs (film), 96
Vibrators, 143–44, 148
Victoria's Secret, 113
Videotapes
    learning from, 67
    for self-love, 146
    See also Films
Virginity
    men losing, 15
    women losing, 16, 33–34
Visualization exercises, 155
Visual mantra, 35–37
Viva Las Vegas (film), 102
Vixens, 101–2, 104
    See also Sexpots
Votaw, Melanie, 41
Vulva, sex words for, 129–30

Ward, Rachel, 104
Wardrobe, 68
    discomfort of, 113–14

of dominatrixes, 88, 90, 113
of femmes fatale, 73, 74
for the novice exhibitionist, 112–13
of sex kittens and Lolitas, 104
of slutty girls, 103–4
Welch, Raquel, 69, 96
Weld, Tuesday, 74
West, Mae, 6, 10, 26, 98, 100, 103, 123
Wet and Dry Aquassager (sex toy), 151
Who Framed Roger Rabbit? (film), 103
Wildfire (S&M club), 92
Will Success Spoil Rock Hunter? (film),
    103
Women
    ejaculation of, 109–10
    fantasies of, 17
    genetic programming of, 12
    initiating men to sex, 15–17
    liberated, 10, 20
    and mating, 12, 13
    orgasms of, 16
    power of, 3, 4, 12, 13, 17, 27, 94, 173
    pubococcygeus (PC) muscle, 155–56,
        157–61
    sexual physiology of, 156
Women's Essential Sex Tonic
    (aphrodisiac), 168
Women's movement, 9–10
"Wonderful Tonight" (song), 121
Wood, Natalie, 84
Writing, erotic, 39–47, 127
Wydra, Nancilee
    Designing Your Happiness, 138
    Feng Shui: Book of Cures, 138
    Feng Shui for Singles, 138

X-rated films, 14, 146

Yoga, Tantric, 178
Yohimbe, 167, 168, 170
"You Can Leave Your Hat On" (song), 121